THE WAY THROUGH

The Way Through

*Trauma Responsive Care for Intellectual and
Developmental Disability Professionals*

Lara Palay, LISW-S

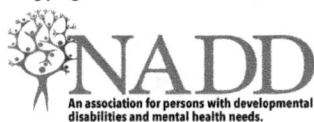

NADD
An association for persons with developmental
disabilities and mental health needs.

321 Wall Street, Kingston, N.Y., 12401

ISBN 979-8-9853366-0-3 (paperback)
ISBN 979-8-9853366-1-0 (e-book)

Cover and book design by Mark Sullivan
Author photo by Jen Hearn

Printed in the United States of America

table of contents

Foreword ... *ix*

Introduction: The Angel and the Waiting Room ... *xi*

Chapter One: Intellectual/Developmental Disabilities, Dual Diagnosis, and Trauma ... *1*

Chapter Two: Trauma 101 ... *11*

Chapter Three: Brain Basics (including We Don't Always Know What We Think We Know or How I Got Everything about Your Brain Wrong) ... *31*

Chapter Four: Trauma Responsive Care: Safe, Connected, and In Control ... *51*

Chapter Five: Starting with the Right Person ... *65*

Chapter Six: The CALMER Skills ... *83*

Chapter Seven: The Main Points in This Book ... *97*

Conclusion: The Way Through ... *101*

Chapter Eight: Questions ... *107*

Acknowledgments ... *119*

Index ... *123*

Source Material and Recommended Reading ... *127*

Endnotes ... *129*

This book is dedicated to
Jim Lantz, Ph.D.
and
Elizabeth "Liz" Ely Palay, MSW, Ph.D.
May their memories be as a blessing.

foreword
....

The first time I saw Lara Palay, she was presenting at a conference for the National Association for the Dually Diagnosed in Charlotte, N.C. I was struck with the clarity and force she had when presenting. And her topic was riveting: trauma and its effect on mental health. I made sure I got to know her! Now she has written a book with the same clarity and force. It is an important read.

Not only does *The Way Through* clarify many of the complex mechanisms of trauma in simple, easily understood terms, it also provides useful tools. Lara's explanation of Trauma Responsive Care is an excellent guideline for working with people with intellectual disabilities who have experienced trauma. She also provides a framework for those working directly with people with intellectual disabilities through her CALMER approach. Her understanding that we, ourselves, are the most critical tool we have when working with people with intellectual disabilities and mental health challenges goes a long way. Her approach is not only theoretical, she gives us the concrete tools for ongoing application as well.

It is past time that we who are providing supports for people with intellectual disabilities and mental health challenges learn about trauma and the critical components of healing. Lara's book is an excellent assist in this endeavor. Her stories, insights, and tools illuminate the way forward for those us of working in this field.

Karyn Harvey, Ph.D.

The Angel and the Waiting Room

A True Story

When it was the early Nineties, I was in my early twenties. I got hired part-time at a local crisis shelter for teenagers. I loved that job, especially after my previous gigs in college. These had included things like sitting alone and bored at a dry cleaner, endless tray-schlepping and dish-washing in a cafeteria, and once, memorably, checking IDs and bouncing drunks at a local bar (but that's for the next book).

I liked working at the shelter because I was interested in listening to the young people's stories. I enjoyed solving problems and I showed some talent for it. It paid okay, most of my coworkers were my age, and the hours were flexible. I know now that I also liked the *feeling* of doing that job. I was proud that I was good at it, and it seemed like my helping others meant I was a noble person.

Then I was hired for their new program: housing for older teens with more serious emotional problems. We had one young man named James.[1] He'd had a tough life in his seventeen years, but that didn't change the fact that he could be a giant pain. He complained nonstop and stirred up gossip and drama with the other residents. He avoided doing chores and had to be nagged constantly to go to his appointments or take his medication. Nothing was ever right, no one was ever doing enough to help, and he was never, ever treated fairly—according to him. James was not my favorite, and I didn't look forward to working with him, but I managed to be polite to him. One Saturday night he did the thing he was known for: He got upset about something some other resident had said to him (I no longer have any idea what it was, if I ever did know), and then, running out into the courtyard of our building, he announced at the top of his lungs that he was going to kill himself. He didn't do anything to physically harm himself, but the threat was enough. This of course made the whole place go, to use the clinical term, *completely nuts*. We called the squad, word raced around the unit, and the other residents joyfully crowded around to yell encouragement or goad James on. He screamed obscenities at the staff in Spanish and flailed his arms around while the EMTs tried to evaluate him. At this point the neighbors came out to see what was so exciting, and I figured the police could only be next. After that it would be the news crews and *after that*, I decided, we'd all be fired (which, at that moment, didn't sound so bad). While my coworkers struggled to calm the other teenagers and get them back inside, I got nominated to accompany James to the emergency room.

Once there, we were shunted off to the mental health section, where we sat in massive, deliberately-chosen-because-they're-too-heavy-to-throw wooden chairs in a small room with cracked linoleum tile on the floor. We waited. By now James was chatty, cheerfully complaining about how long it was all taking. I gritted my teeth while I found snacks for him from a vending machine and he watched the TV bolted to the wall. I knew every suicide threat had to be taken seriously, but he certainly seemed to be making the most of the excitement and change of scenery. The only other person with us in that dingy waiting room was a stocky man with buzz-cut grey hair, in his late sixties. He sat behind a too-heavy-to-throw wooden desk with nothing on it, doing word searches in a puzzle book. It seemed likely that monitoring us was his retirement job. He looked as though his former career had been as a bank security guard or maybe a probation officer. I got more and more irritated with James as the minutes and then hours ticked by, long past when my shift should have ended. *This is my Saturday night*, I thought. *Awesome.*

Finally, a nurse came to take James to an examination room and I waited to see if he would be admitted or not. After James left with her, the guard shifted in his seat and looked up from his book. "These kids today," he began, and I braced myself for a speech about the declining standards of our schools, or maybe the evils of rap music. *Oh man*, I thought. *Here we go.*

"These kids today. They sure have a hard time."

He blinked at me and then calmly went back to his puzzles. I sat frozen in my giant wooden chair. This big, lumbering-looking man had been kinder about James in a few seconds than I had been that whole grudging evening. Maybe kinder about him than I'd *ever* been. He reminded me, whether he intended to or not, that *James was, in fact, a kid. And he was having a hard time.*

Eventually they brought James out and we went back to the shelter. By then it was too late to go out with my friends as I'd planned. As I drove home, I felt numb and agitated at the same time. There's no way to say this without sounding corny, so I won't try; I'll just tell you how it was. That one small comment from the security guard made me feel as if my heart had cracked open a little inside my chest.

I can't say that after that day, working with James suddenly became a delight. It did not. He was still demanding and obstinate and could make a huge nuisance of himself. None of that magically changed. But I felt softer about him. I could see his pain and damage so much more clearly now. I could see that at any given moment, he was doing the best he could—even if sometimes his best was still pretty damned annoying.

You know how this story ends: After that evening, my relationship with James changed. This new way of looking at James let me be genuinely caring with him, rather than going through the motions in a secret bad mood. I became one of the staff who could reach him and sometimes talk him down from the dizzying heights of his ridiculous dramatics. The drama, the exaggeration—all of that *was* ridiculous. But for the first time, I could appreciate that James, himself, was not ridiculous. He was sad and confused and angry and hurt. He sensed how alienating he could be. He knew his best ideas for handling problems were basically terrible and usually made things worse. I think he sometimes felt he messed up everything he touched. Now I could see this pattern he was stuck in and, more importantly, how lonely and frustrating it was for him. The simplest way to say it, I guess, is that now I fully felt his humanity. Maybe to an outsider the way I dealt with him wouldn't have looked that different; it's not like I screamed or said mean things to him before all this happened. But I knew that on the inside, everything about how I was with him had shifted. *It wasn't about changing him—it was about changing me.*

It turns out the security guard's kindness changed everything about how I work, forever. I've gained a lot of knowledge since that night when I sat, bored and annoyed, in the waiting room with the clunky furniture and the grubby floor. I've gone to school to study mental illness and gotten years of experience doing psychotherapy with a wide variety of clients. I've taught graduate students about the clinical aspects of the most appalling things that can happen to a human being. I've shown them how to offer help and consolation for someone enduring grief, horror, and despair. I lecture to audiences about how trauma works and what our brains and bodies do when we're afraid. I can cite research and studies. I think that as I've gotten older, I've become more observant and perceptive. But I still reach back to that moment in the waiting room whenever I'm exasperated with a client, a supervisee, or a student. The compassion of that security guard's remark opens me up to try to see *what is actually going on with this person*. Remembering that, my heart softens—sometimes just a little—and I can see that person more clearly. I change myself, and my ability to work with them changes. Skills, knowledge, planning, teamwork—of course these are still, and always will be, important when we're trying to help people. But if I don't work with myself first, I'm of little use to anybody, including me.

In the decades since James, I've thought a lot about that guard. If angels exist, I think maybe he was one. He appeared just at the time he was needed, taking the unassuming form of a bulky man behind an empty desk to say exactly the right words, to point out the thing that was true that I hadn't been seeing—to prod me gently to be kind. I sometimes imagine that after we walked out that night, he just vanished, one of those "people" who show up in disguise, playing a role for us for the time we're with them and then winking out of physical existence as soon as we've left, their job done.[2] When I was younger, I assumed the angel was there for James. Now I think maybe he was in that waiting room for me, to help me be a little better than I was.

This Book Is for You

For Direct Services Professionals (DSPs), past and present
Some of you took this job in the field of intellectual and developmental disabilities (I/DD) because it fit your needs: the pay, the hours, or maybe the location. Some of you chose your work for other reasons. You may have a sibling, cousin, or child with a disability, or you know

someone who works in this field and loves what they do. Whatever the reason you're in your job, this book will touch on the heart of being sensitive and present for the people you work with. It will make you better at your job. Whatever your reasons for what you do, this book is for you.

For managers

Why do you supervise staff? You may have moved into your role after being a DSP yourself. You may have experience in other areas (like mine in mental health) and found your way to the developmental disabilities field. Maybe this is a role you took on to help your agency as it figures out staffing, and it's just one of many other responsibilities you have right now. Whatever the route you took, this book is for you, too.

For clinicians, psychologists, and other specialists

Why are you a clinician? This is a question I could have asked myself in many of my jobs, and the answer would have taken days. Doing clinical work is demanding, tiring, and exciting. For me, there is no other job in the world that satisfies me as much. If you work with clients who have disabilities, the challenges and rewards are even bigger. If you would like to understand more about trauma and the way it affects your clients, this book can help. If you are a skilled trauma therapist already but you need to explain trauma in clear, compassionate language to the people around your client, this book is for you.

NO MORE ENFORCERS, NO MORE BABYSITTERS

I've talked with hundreds of people in audiences all over the United States and in other countries. When I ask them, "When do you like your job working with people with disabilities?" no one ever says, "When I get to enforce a rule!" or "I just love being someone's babysitter!"

When I ask them, "How do you know you've had a good day at work?" they always say the same things:

I like knowing I helped someone.

I like knowing my individual had a good day.

I like supporting my staff through a tough situation.

I like making someone smile.

I like helping my individual reach a new goal.

I like helping my staff do a job they feel good about.

Nobody ever raises their hand and says, "I want to be yelling and frustrated and exerting total control over people at all times."

If you came to this work for a job, this book will make you better at what you do and make your job more interesting, less stressful, and more rewarding. If you came to this work with a sense of love, mission, and purpose (or found these things along the way), this book will help you realize that purpose. Very few people sign up to work with people because they want to be a babysitter or jail warden, but all too often when we're dealing with an individual who, from our point of view, is acting strangely or making things difficult, we turn into jailers. We focus on control instead of understanding, and we try to change them rather than adjusting ourselves. If they're agitated or upset, we take it as a reflection on us or a personal attack, and we decide that, by God, we're going to *make it stop*. If they're shut-down and passive, we give up on engaging them. *Ugh, what's the point?* And we become babysitters.

In this book, we'll work together to understand how trauma often is something that is part (if not most) of what is making some of our individuals "act strangely." I'll cover how much traumatic stress and other mental health issues are a part of our individuals' lives and what happens when we miss it. For those of you who are familiar with trauma, I hope it will be a good review, and for those for whom trauma is a new area, I hope it will be a useful introduction. We'll look at exactly what is happening in someone's brain when they are fearful or living out a past trauma. I'll talk about why most of what you've been taught to do in those situations not only doesn't help but might be making it worse. Then, I'll explain what *does* help: Trauma Responsive Care.

Trauma Responsive Care (TRC) is the next step beyond trauma-informed care. Being informed is where we start with any issue, so it's a necessary beginning. But trauma-informed care models don't tell us much about what we should actually do when we're with a trauma-tized person, or how to do it. Trauma Responsive Care takes you from *awareness* to *responsiveness*. TRC can help you do things differently with someone who has been traumatized. This won't be because I give you some magic formula to change the person you're working with, whether it's an individual, a staff person, or a colleague. It will be because you approach things differently. As I did with James, you change yourself.

After introducing the concepts of TRC (safe, connected, and in control), I'll take you through a series of steps called the CALMER Skills. These can help you to get yourself into the right frame of mind to do things that help your individual, rather than things that don't. We'll work together on understanding what happens to your sensations, emotions, and thoughts when someone is reliving a trauma, and how to keep yourself grounded and aware. When I say we'll work together, it's because there are simple questions and exercises at the end of the book. These are your chance to bring your own experiences and insight to this process.

If you are a supervisor or a manager, you might be working directly with individuals, too. But even if you focus solely on supporting staff, you need to be able to do the things in this book. You may be the first (or only) person staff can reliably turn to when they are being challenged. Your ability to understand how human beings react to stress and fear doesn't apply just to the individuals you serve. Noticing when a staff person, family member, colleague, or yourself is triggered or locked into a power struggle makes you the most powerful person in that situation.

There are some tools in this book, like the CALMER Skills and the Golden Square (attunement, attachment, attention, and adjustment). These can help you understand what's going on inside you when you are dealing with another person, so you can figure out how to work with your inner experience effectively. These approaches may help with situations in your everyday personal life, too. I hope they do. But remember, you can use what feels comfortable and skip anything that feels too emotionally intense. In my trainings, I usually don't take people through an inventory of their own traumatic experiences or personal history. That can get way too intrusive, fast. However, some of the stories and ideas in this book might bring up sensations, feelings, or memories from your life—maybe some that are pleasant and some not so pleasant. This is normal. If the stories help you to connect to something that makes the information more vivid and memorable, great. If anything becomes too stressful, then just skip that part. If you find yourself consistently feeling worried, stressed, or disconnected, it's a good idea to talk to someone supportive. You may want to work with a therapist to understand and integrate your experiences. Make sure your agency has employee assistance or mental health resources for referrals for your staff, as well.

If this book helps you to see a little more of the humanity or the pain or the fear inside the person you're working with, then it might change how you look at them, the way I was changed that night at the hospital. It might help you, when you use the information and tools in this book, to reach that other person in a new way that works. I hope some of the things we'll talk about here will appear in your mind to open things up for you, making things easier than they were, the way my security guard—if that's what he really was—showed up to help me all those years ago. You carry the key to opening that small, grungy waiting room we've all been in before—when we're locked into anger and frustration, or trying to move others out of it. Maybe that's the room an individual has spent a lot of time in, literally or figuratively. Some of the people we support have been trapped in their reactions, out of step with what's happening around them, for a long time. You can help everyone involved to walk out. Understanding and working differently with trauma, in everyday interactions, really can be a key to healing it. Your individuals, your staff, your agency—whatever role you play at work, they need you, and their lives will be all the better because *you* are there, in that room with them. That is the beginning of the way through.

chapter one

Intellectual and Developmental Disabilities, Dual Diagnosis, and Trauma

Actual things I have heard said about people with intellectual and developmental disabilities:

> *"He was beaten by his dad when he was two and had been in three different placements by the time he was five, but he doesn't remember any of it, so I don't think he was traumatized."*

> *"Our individual's mother died five months ago and she's still asking about her. When will she forget about her mom?"*

> *"My client was raped twenty years ago, and he brings it up every month when I meet with him. Why does he still need to talk about it? I think he should let it go."*

If you ask someone in mental health who their toughest clients are, many of them will tell you it's the people on their caseload who have an intellectual or developmental disability. The others might not think of it, because we in the mental health world sometimes focus on substance abuse and forget the *other* "dual diagnosis"—mental illness and I/DD. That's our mistake, by the way, because while we work hard to deal with co-occurring substance issues, we often get disabilities wrong, especially with folks with "borderline intellectual functioning" who may not qualify for much I/DD support but usually have our worst mental health services outcomes. If you ask someone in the I/DD world who *their* toughest folks are, they usually don't make the same mistake. They'll invariably say, "People with dual diagnoses," and *they* mean I/DD and mental illness. For this book, we're going to focus on one of the most common and most misunderstood mental illnesses (or *injury*, as I sometimes talk about it): trauma.

To talk about trauma in the people we serve, we should start with the kinds of traumas people experience and how often they may be exposed to that risk.

The National Core Indicators, information about I/DD services shared among states in the U.S., say that thirty percent of people with intellectual or developmental disabilities served in this country have a mood disorder, twenty-seven percent have issues with anxiety, and twenty-eight percent have a behavioral disorder. Fifty-four percent take at least one medication usually prescribed for a mental illness.[3] If I have an intellectual or developmental disorder, I may be up to four times more likely to have a mental health issue than someone in the general population.[4]

Trauma is likely to be one of the obstacles they face. Anywhere from fifty to ninety percent of the general adult population will experience a traumatic event in their lifetime.[5]

According to the U.S. Department of Justice statistics, in 2011, nearly three out of a thousand people with a disability experienced rape or a sexual assault. Thirty-six out of a thousand experienced some type of assault.[6] Researchers estimate that only one in thirty cases of sexual abuse of a person with I/DD gets reported.[7] Any social problem you can think of, from poverty to disease, is more likely to happen to someone if they also have a disability, and trauma is at the top of that list.[8] It's estimated that sixty to ninety percent of people with intellectual disabilities may suffer from trauma.[9]

We used to think that if you had a developmental disability, you couldn't also have mental illness. When I started working with the Ohio Department of Developmental Disabilities in 2009, there were still doctors and psychiatrists practicing (most of that generation now retired, thankfully) who said that kind of thing. Now it's common knowledge in our field that having I/DD actually makes you *more* vulnerable to having a mental illness.[10]

When I began learning about dual diagnosis, some of the same diagnoses given to people with I/DD came up over and over. Here are some of the disorders with which people with I/DD in the U.S. typically are diagnosed:[11]

- Depression, bipolar disorder
- Borderline personality disorder
- Anxiety, obsessive-compulsive disorder (OCD)
- Attention deficit hyperactivity disorder (ADHD), oppositional defiant disorder, and intermittent explosive disorder
- Schizophrenia and schizoaffective disorder

With my background in trauma, what struck me as I was learning this new-to-me world of "dual diagnosis" is that all of those diagnoses *are also common misdiagnoses of trauma*.[12] I don't mean just in people who also have a disability. I mean for everybody—soldiers, survivors of rape and assault, people in domestically violent homes. In the mental health world, we've known for decades that trauma can look like any one of these disorders at a given moment. It was said in our field that the average person with Post-Traumatic Stress Disorder (PTSD) would have gotten four other diagnoses before someone landed on the right one; hopefully that's not still the case, but if you've ever known someone with trauma, that might sound familiar still.

I explain to my graduate students that trauma is like an octopus. (I guess in this metaphor, we're in the "ocean of mental health problems.") Depending on which tentacle you've got ahold of, trauma can look like depression, schizophrenia, and personality disorders—one tentacle reaching into low mood, another into the distorted perceptions of dissociation, yet another into an unstable pattern of grasping for, yet hating, closeness. So, my earlier comment isn't a slap at diagnosticians. It's easy to see how hard it can be to figure out what you're dealing with, depending on what you're looking at in a person.

As clinicians, we learned to see one of these diagnoses—especially bipolar, borderline, and ADHD—and look for trauma. Much of the time, in my experience, we found it. It could be concurrent; you can certainly have PTSD *and* schizophrenia at the same time. But too often trauma had been missed entirely; once that trauma was dealt with, the symptoms of the "other disorder" mysteriously vanished.

THE FIRST PROBLEM: HOW WE SEE OTHERS

If I sound angry about this, it's just because I am. Misdiagnosing trauma as something else can have real and devastating consequences. One problem is that sometimes we diagnose people based on what they look like, how we feel about them, or what we think we know about their lives—*not on what is actually going on with them.* We know from piles of studies[13, 14]—I've chosen to cite just a few—that if, for example, you are a Black boy in this country and you are struggling with something, you are more likely to be given a behavioral diagnosis (ADHD, oppositional defiant disorder, disruptive behavior disorder).[15] But in my experience, a white child (especially a girl) with the same symptoms is more likely to be given a diagnosis of an adjustment or mood disorder (situational stresses, anxiety, depression). Any social worker, psychologist, or other mental health professional is a human being, with all the biases we humans sometimes have. It's easy to see how some people appear to us to be "sad" (sympathetic, nonthreatening, appealing to helpers) and some people appear "bad" ("not behaving right," scary, problems that need to be fixed).

I believe the same thing can happen with developmental disabilities, and now we have to add another layer of potential bias. Mental health problems in someone with a disability can go unseen and untreated because people with intellectual and developmental disabilities are vulnerable to "diagnostic overshadowing." Stephen Reiss at Ohio State University coined this term after researching how doctors treat people with I/DD.[16] He found that a diagnosis of a developmental disability tends to overshadow anything else that might be going on with an individual. For example, let's say I'm banging my head or clenching my teeth. This gets explained away by saying, "Oh, Lara just does that" because I have I/DD. My staff and family might not realize the banging and clenching are signs of pain from a raging sinus infection. Other explanations aren't considered because the disability answers everything. It simply never occurs to anyone to check more carefully. If they did, they might find out that I'm banging my head because I have painful sinus pressure and the counterpressure feels good, or I'm scared (or triggered) and hurting myself to distract from my fear. Reiss found it can work the same way in the other direction, too: attributing *nothing* to having a developmental disability—I'm acting the way I am because I'm "crazy," or I'm trying to be difficult or manipulative. The answer is we have to take bias into account, and we *have* to look more closely than just basing assumptions on the surface of a person. Put these complications together—all the confusing aspects of trauma, biases inherent in our culture, and diagnostic over-shadowing—and it's easy to see why trauma still goes unrecognized so often in people with I/DD.

What do we do if we think someone with I/DD might have a mental health problem? In the mental health world, meds and therapy together are the "gold standard" for how to treat most common disorders like anxiety, depression, and trauma. But in the I/DD world, meds and behavior plans are the first and only options many people think of. We know we have a problem with overmedication of people with I/DD. There's also a lot of off-label prescribing.[17] The NCI project documented a ten percent gap in the number of people taking these meds versus the number of people with diagnoses that suggest they need that medication. Nationally, that adds up to thousands of people.[18] It's hard not to conclude that at least some of those people are being given medication based on how disruptive they are, rather than on medical considerations (more on this later). It's hard not to see *that* as an attempt to address (that is: control) behavior through medications. At high enough levels, we call that chemical restraint.

Having said all that, now I have to balance it a bit. It's important to remember that some medications are developed for one kind of problem, but then doctors find out it treats other issues as well. Viagra was originally prescribed to treat high blood pressure. So was Tenex, and now it's used to help stabilize moods. This "off-label" use is common; over time we learn more about what a drug does in different people. The problem, in my opinion, is that this makes it easy to operate in a grey area where people are given meds without a diagnosis that suggests they need them—and that suggests that some-times we are *medicating behavior.*

THE SECOND PROBLEM: HOW WE SEE OURSELVES

"... [T]here is almost nothing harder for humans than to look in the mirror and honestly say, '[I am] the problem.'" [19]

What's left if we don't medicate someone? We target behavior alone.

To a mental health person, the I/DD field sometimes seems like it's stuck in the past.[20] All too often I hear about cases that are being viewed, however compassionately, from a purely behavioral standpoint: Sierra is doing A and we want her to do B. When Sierra starts doing B, case closed. If she's non-speaking and she's doing puzzling, weird stuff, staff want to address it. This is true especially if it's dangerous. I know how urgent it is to get Sierra to stop, and if punishments and rewards can quickly shape her behavior in a better direction, that's quite seductive. I get the allure. There's nothing wrong with teaching Sierra to act differently. The problem is that it's so easy to leave it there—as long as Sierra is acting "better," no one is going to ask questions. But we need to ask who Sierra is and how she can *be* better, not just *behave* better. And if Sierra doesn't start acting better—and quick!—it's easy to see how someone can feel threatened or angry. I'll discuss this in more detail later, but how people make us feel *about ourselves* affects how we treat them. If I can't get you to "behave" when I want you to, or if I like helping people to "feel better" and I can't get you to stop feeling sad or scared or mad, you can undermine *how I feel about myself*. How I feel I'm doing my job. How my coworkers or my boss or the other residents see me. When I start to feel bad about myself or about the job I'm doing, it's hard for me to blame myself for that, but it's easy to blame *you*. And that's the moment when, whether I'm aware of it or not, bad things can happen.

In these kinds of situations, we need to be asking questions beyond "How can we make this stop?" Understanding trauma will help us do that.

One thing I think is valuable about a mental health perspective is that we often view mental illness as curable. When it's not, in the case of a major persistent mental illness like schizophrenia, we try to get that patient into remission or at least control the symptoms so they aren't causing the client insurmountable problems. This is one of the biggest "cultural" differences I found between mental health and the I/DD world. A developmental disability, by definition, is something that someone is born with, or it comes from an injury that hurt that person's ability to develop in typical ways. The effects are lifelong; while people can definitely see improvement in how they cope, I/DD professionals don't expect their individual's condition to be cured or go into remission. This means the individual will probably need some form of support all their lives, "from the cradle to the grave."

Resolving or managing mental illness usually is time-limited. Many people with a mental illness will have the illness resolve and never need treatment again; some people will use medication and therapy on and off for their whole lives; and some people need constant monitoring, medication, and support. But the overall model is to treat and release; we refer to it as "recovery and resilience."

For I/DD professionals, this can be puzzling and frustrating. You finally get mental health services for your dually diagnosed individual, they make progress, and then you're told by the mental health center, "Okay, we reached our goals. We're closing the case." You assumed the services would be in place forever, or at least for a long time. People who have dual diagnoses often need both acute treatment for their mental health issue and support for the disability throughout their lives.

We might think about trauma as being a doorway, a midway point between these two expectations. Someone who suffers a single-event trauma but had a stable childhood and no other significant emotional or physiological stress may recover completely, sometimes even without treatment.[21, 22] Someone who experienced severe, long-lasting trauma, especially if their childhood was also stressful, might very well be dealing with some aftereffects their whole lives. When we work with people who have an intellectual or developmental disability *and* trauma, we can take both approaches. We can work toward recovery *and* plan for ongoing support.

chapter two
....

Trauma 101

"Trauma is a disease of not being able to be here."

—Pierre Janet

This is the most elegant definition I've ever heard about the problem with trauma. People struggling with trauma can miss out on so much of their own lives, spending time either "frozen or frantic" inside, profoundly out of step with what is going on around them.

I think they're also isolated by what other people don't know about trauma. One of the most important things people get wrong when dealing with someone with trauma is this impatient feeling we have that if the person would just *get over it,* everything would be better. As Bessel van der Kolk says,

> In fact, the past is the past and the only thing that matters is what happens right now. And what is trauma is the residue that a past event leaves in your own sensory experiences in your body and it's not that event out there that becomes intolerable but the physical sensations with which you live that become intolerable and you will do anything to make them go away.[23]

Trauma isn't just in our memories—it's in our brains and bodies, here in the present.

Trauma is any experience or series of experiences that make you feel you are going to die or be emotionally "wiped out" or annihilated. Van der Kolk explains it simply: "An experience becomes traumatic when the human organism becomes overwhelmed and reacts with helplessness and paralysis."[24]

Let's look at how something becomes traumatic. Traumatic events change the brain and body in ways we are just learning to understand. Trauma is like a fire that damages a sprinkler system in a building. Our brain's alarm system is thrown off, so now the alarm goes off too easily or fails to go off at all. Traumatized people over- or underreact to threats (real or imagined). An example is the story a former boss of mine told me years ago:

*While working on a domestic violence hotline, I took a call from a woman. She sounded composed and I began as I always did, by asking her, "Are you in a safe place right now?" She said yes, she was, and we went on with the conversation. Maybe half an hour into the call, she mentioned offhandedly that her husband was pacing outside her door with a loaded gun. Shocked, I asked her why she'd told me earlier that that she was "in a safe place." She answered in a surprised tone of voice, saying, "Well, he's not **in the room with me**."*

This woman's sense of danger had been shifted by her traumatic experiences, so her alarm system wasn't set off by her husband stalking around with a gun in the next room—a situation another person probably would find terrifying.

Trauma raises hormone levels, especially the stress hormone cortisol. This can be physically devastating; there are more receptors for this chemical than for any other neurotransmitter in the body.

This increase in stress can last for decades. Our brain's limbic system, which filters out irrelevant information, becomes "programmed for stress." This shift can cause chronic overfocusing and hypervigilance or a feeling of numbness and detachment from life. Some people alternate between these two states—freaked out or checked out—never resting in calm alertness.

A promising way we are thinking about and treating trauma is Steven Porges's polyvagal theory.[25] We'll talk more about the vagus nerve in the next chapter, Brain Basics. For now, this model is a good way to introduce the three levels of activation or "arousal" in our brain and body.

Our brains and bodies operate on one of three levels:

Social "engagement" zone (awake, calm, alert for unusual sensation or minor threat): You're calm in your environment and then something happens. Maybe there is an unfamiliar sight or sound. The reason it's hard to sleep in a new place is that your brain hasn't sorted out which sounds are safe and which ones might not be. You startle awake at every creak. Once you're used to being where you are, your brain automatically filters out the normal sounds (the hum of the air conditioner switching on) but wakes you up for something that is unfamiliar (steps on the stairs). My cats can race wildly around our house at night and it rarely wakes me up, but I would react to the slightest noise when one of my teenaged sons would try to sneak in late at night. When we are calm and aware, our heart rate is normal, our breathing is regular, and our attention is relaxed. Trauma therapists sometimes refer to this state as a "window of tolerance,"[26] a range for noticing and reacting appropriately. We can tolerate what's going on around us. This is sometimes called the "engagement zone." We can engage with the environment in a relaxed and easy way. Imagine you are sitting outside and you hear a commotion in the trees above you. You glance up, paying attention to the new sound. You see that it's a squirrel rustling around and your brain quickly decides "not a threat" and you go back to what you were doing. You probably don't immediately start screaming in terror or collapse in a faint on the ground.

When we are in our window of tolerance and we're talking to someone, we can engage with them appropriately. We're alert but relaxed, standing at a comfortable distance for whatever culture we're from—not too close, not too far away. We're as "social"—introverted or extroverted—as we normally are with people. We may be curious about them and let them know things about us. Even if an issue comes up between us, we address it and try to fix it. The threat, if one exists, is manageable and our body doesn't get activated.

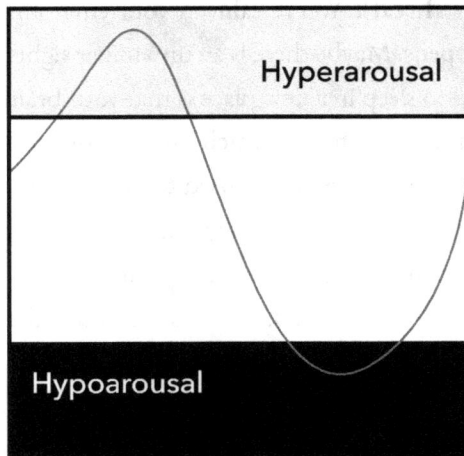

Adrenalized, sympathetic state (moderate threat; ready to take action with fight, flight, freeze, or fawn): Something has happened in the environment (a loud noise, an angry face) that lets us know we may be facing a threat, and our body gets ready to go to work. Our brain signals our body to release the stress hormones cortisol and adrenaline. Our heart rate speeds up, and maybe we feel shaky as our body prepares to run or to fight the threat.

- *Fight:* We are aggressive and may lash out physically to overcome a threat.
- *Flight:* We are ready to run away from the threat.
- *Freeze:* This can look like helplessness and *collapse* (which we'll get to in a moment), but it isn't. Freezing is *stillness at a high state of tension.* The best example of this might be a rabbit that runs out in front of your car. The rabbit is stock-still, but it bolts away as soon as you swerve past it. It's active in its survival attempt by freezing—motionless for the moment, then springing into action.
- *Fawn:* This has also been called "tend and befriend." To "fawn" in this context means to excessively flatter and fuss over someone. This survival reaction is to *move closer to the threat* to neutralize it. Placating, appeasing, smiling, or acting seductively may make a threatening, angry person calm down and no longer pose a danger to us. Anyone might go into a state of *fawning,* but in many cultures, women have been socialized to behave this way already, so we may see this reaction more often in female-identifying people.

Collapse, dissociation (serious or prolonged threat; unable to challenge or escape): At this third level, the threat is so great that we can only shut down. This might look like a relaxed, limp, folded-in posture or vacant facial expression. Bessel van der Kolk notes that we go into a collapsed state if we are physically unable to escape the danger (for example, trapped in a crushed car after an accident) or if our previous attempts to escape the danger have failed. This goes toward explaining "learned helplessness," the state in which a creature has tried repeatedly to avoid something painful or fearful and cannot, so it doesn't even try anymore. A collapsed state can be not only outward stillness but also comparatively little activity in the brain.[27] In *collapse*, we are motionless, but unlike *freeze*, collapse is a de-energized state. If *fight-flight-freeze-fawn* are states in which we're highly activated for safety, like being in a house with the fire alarms blaring and the lights flashing, *collapse* is like being in a cold, dark house with no electricity and a locked door. Safety comes from locking down or not being present. In contrast to the rabbit that is frozen and ready to run, when we are in *collapse* we are a rabbit that's limp in the jaws of a wolf. The rabbit's muscles are slack, and even if the wolf drops him, he might just lie there. He's passive, waiting for the next thing to happen.

This shutdown can also create *dissociation*. Dissociation simply means "things that are usually connected are now disconnected." When people are emotionally dissociated, they'll describe themselves as feeling cold, numb, empty, or bored. Some of my clients have said that when they dissociate, they feel they're not in their bodies anymore—physical (or perceptual) dissociating. *"It's as if I'm floating on the ceiling and looking at what's happening, like it's happening to someone else."* When it's extreme, dissociation can cause people to lose track of big chunks of time or even feel they contain other people (or fragments of people) inside them. This is now called Dissociative Identity Disorder[28] but may be more familiar to you as Multiple Personality Disorder.

In more common cases, dissociation is often a disconnect between thinking and feeling. I worked with refugees who had gone through unimaginable trauma before they asked for asylum in the U.S. In a session, someone would start telling the story of their torture and abuse, without being asked about it (I would *never* have asked them to discuss the details of their traumatic events, especially early in therapy). Each time, I noticed that the person told the story like hitting a "play" button on a recording. Robotically, they recited horrible events with little or no emotion on their faces or in their voices. Sometimes I had to work hard not to cry, hearing what had happened to them. But they talked as if they were repeating a list of groceries. This is *dissociation*—in this case, separating the emotions from what happened. A psychologist I saw at a trauma training (who used the example of the houses I mentioned earlier) said it simply: "Dissociation makes the unbearable bearable."

Our nervous system has two goals: survive and then thrive. Our brain and body will do whatever it takes to meet these goals. The brain will make this work as well as it can over time by creating a set point, whichever level of activation is most frequently used. Child psychiatrist Bruce Perry, an expert in childhood trauma, says "the state becomes a trait."[29] This means that whatever state our brain spends the most time in (calm; fight/flight; dissociated/shut down) will be more and more familiar. This familiar brain state can look like someone's whole personality, which is why trauma that has been missed can create daily problems for the people we serve. You might be told, "Oh, Lara's always aggressive and irritable; that's just who she is." But the truth is that my brain is in fight-or-flight mode *most of the time*. It also means my brain's threshold for going into that state gets lower and lower; in other words, it takes less to set me off into that fight-or-flight reaction. It may well take longer and longer for me to get back into my window of tolerance. My relationships (or lack of them), my support plans, and my staffing all may reflect this aggressive, irritable person people see, but they mask my true self. I think that's what Pierre Janet was talking about in that quote at the beginning of this chapter—that the real tragedy of trauma is that it can rob us of the lives we were meant to live. It keeps us from being the people we really are.

Like all the states we've discussed so far, collapse and dissociating are normal reactions to danger, built into brains. Some people will progress in order through these levels of reacting; others will jump to a stronger reaction like collapse right away. Bessel van der Kolk says stressful events are even more likely to be traumatizing if we are physically trapped or held still. That means restraint during a flashback may make the traumatic damage even worse.

None of the reactions we've talked about here is wrong, but they can create problems. One serious effect of untreated trauma is that these reactions can keep happening long after the threat is over, stopping us from handling new threats effectively. Some people will wildly overreact to a minor surprise. Others may underreact to a real danger. Some people who have lived through sexual assault, for example, will find that when someone around them is behaving inappropriately or dangerously, they (the survivor) will go into a collapsed, shut-down, passive state. This numbness, like that of the woman in my boss's story, might make it hard for the survivor to speak up, set a boundary, get help, or leave. A new assault can happen then and they are traumatized all over again. Dissociation can disable our defense systems. *To be clear, that would NOT make an assault the survivor's fault. Responsibility, as always, falls on the assailant(s) alone and nobody else.*

Traumatized people have trouble integrating new experiences because triggers keep shutting down their present, thinking self, so they get "stuck" neurologically—and psychologically as well.[30] Every new event is tainted by the ongoing past, so they cannot learn from experience, which is why efforts to make change often fail. Suppressing an event in your consciousness and denying the emotions that stem from it take up energy. That leaves none left for living a spontaneous life. (One client described this as "constantly holding the closet door shut.")

Trauma is an injury to the "social brain."

The limbic system, with its emphasis on safety and emotions, has been called by neuroscientists the "social brain." This is always a good reminder to me that we are fundamentally social; it's woven into the fabric of our brains. Interpersonal trauma (which is most of what we see in people with I/DD) can damage how we see ourselves, how we see others, and how we interact with other human beings. It's an injury *from* and *to* other people. It is a relational injury.

When one of my college professors was a young man serving in the Vietnam War, he was a medic. This meant regularly climbing into a helicopter, flying over thick jungle (hoping not to be shot down), landing on a battlefield (praying they didn't set down on a landmine and die instantly), jumping out (again, hoping for no mines), and running out into the field (sometimes under fire) to grab wounded and dying soldiers. He hoped that pieces of them wouldn't come away in his hands when he pulled them off the field. After retrieving the soldiers, he would scramble back into the chopper (hoping that in the thick jungle vegetation they wouldn't hit a branch, breaking off a rotor blade and killing everyone instantly). Heading back to the medical camp, he and the other medics tried desperately to save the wounded men. Many soldiers died on that flight anyway. Sometimes, he said, there were body parts rolling around in the cabin. Always there was blood washing across the floor.

My professor did this every day for a year. Then he came home, got married, and started his career as a therapist and academic. One day, he and his wife decided to go see a movie called *The Deer Hunter*. This was, he would explain to students as he told the story, one of the first graphic, realistic movies about the Vietnam War. As he told it, "One minute, I was a therapist and a professor, sitting next to my wife and watching a movie. The next thing I knew I was crouched in the middle of the aisle screaming 'INCOMING!!' while my wife and an usher tried to drag me out of the theater."

What happened to my professor that night at the movies?

He was triggered.

His brain reacted to seeing the images on screen and it set off an alarm in his brain. When he was in Vietnam, this alarm circuit jump-started the quick reflexes that kept him safe in the war. At the movie, his body was flooded with adrenaline and cortisol, prompting him to jump out of his seat and start screaming, literally before he could think about what he was doing. The need to *fight, flight, freeze,* or *fawn* was so fast and so powerful that it took hold nearly instantaneously. My professor was knocked, violently, out of his window of tolerance. If he had stayed triggered long enough, he might have gone into the deepest part of his survival instinct and *collapsed* or *shut down*.

Not every person who experiences a stressful event is traumatized by it, and not every person who suffers from trauma went through the extremes of war. We know trauma comes in many forms, and how the brain will respond depends on the event and the person. We do know that a terrifying or harmful event caused by another human is often more damaging than impersonal events like a tornado. There's something especially toxic to humans when we're hurt or terrified by other human beings. It cuts deeply into our innate sense that we are valuable to others and that other human beings are a safe source of comfort. We also know the younger a person is when they experience a traumatic event, the more effect it may have on their brain. That is why childhood abuse and neglect can leave such devastation. Trauma may change the safety setpoint in growing brains more than in adult brains that experience similar events.

Traumatic stress is not remembering an event or dwelling on it—it's *reliving* it, without any conscious control over shutting down, exploding, or panicking (the way my professor did). Reliving these events is so confusing, terrifying, and embarrassing that people may have a hard time explaining to others what is going on—they may not even know themselves. Traumatized people will find all sorts of ways not to feel much of anything in order to avoid being triggered. A traumatized person might drink or take drugs, lash out or try to hurt others (sometimes to keep others from hurting them first), overeat or starve themselves, hoard, have random sex, cut themselves, gamble—anything to numb themselves out. People suffering from PTSD often keep doing those things even when those strategies do damage. This is what van der Kolk meant when he said that "you will do anything to make (these sensations) go away."

TRAUMA RESPONSIVE CARE

Why couldn't my professor stop himself from shocking the audience and scaring his wife at the movie? Because the reaction to fear temporarily took over his brain and body. His brain believed he was in danger, just as he was in Vietnam, and his body reacted. He didn't *feel* safe, connected, or in control of himself.

The first step in working with traumatized people is to help them back into their window of tolerance. You must help them calm down if they have been triggered into exploding *or* help them "come back" if they've shut down and dissociated. The best way to help calm and reorient someone who is panicking, lashing out, or shut down with a trauma reaction is to remember the three elements of Trauma Responsive Care: *People need to feel **safe, connected**, and **in control** with you in that moment.* The best way to help someone to recover from trauma means helping that person feel *safe, connected,* and *in control* all the time, not just when they've been triggered.

Reacting vs. Responding

My professor had a reaction to the movie with no time for a response. There is an important difference between a reaction and a response.

A *reaction* happens much faster than a thought. It's the brain getting us away from danger. The brain's escape strategies—running, fighting, or freezing—work well in the face of real danger but not so well in the face of perceived danger. The difference between the body's *reaction* and *response* is the difference between jumping away from a snake lying in wait on the sidewalk and then taking a second look and noticing that the "snake" is actually a stick. The quick reaction keeps us safe, but it is not a sophisticated decision that considers all the important details. Our *reaction* is not in our conscious control. A *response* is what happens when we have an extra second or two to take in more information and think through how we want to behave. *It takes a calmly functioning brain to respond.*

My professor was physically safe in that movie theater, but that didn't matter, because his brain decided he wasn't. These actions can look as out of place and bizarre as my professor must have looked to everyone else in the theater. If you know his story, though, his reaction makes sense. Most of the time we don't know the story behind what originally traumatized a person. The brain learns and strengthens fear reactions, especially if the fear was intense or happened repeatedly. If someone is triggered over and over again, their reaction becomes stronger still. This is how traumatic stress can affect a person decades after the original trauma.

When working with someone who is reacting out of fear, we can get frustrated, scared, or lose our temper. When I talk with audiences, someone will say, "But our consumers *aren't* in danger! We keep our individuals safe!" That's usually true. But we humans react to how safe we *feel*, not how safe we actually *are*. For example, think about flying. Most of us have heard the statistic that we are safer in a plane than we are in our cars driving to the airport. But chances are you feel more nervous on the plane. Why? Because when we are driving our car, we *feel* like we're safer (mostly because we have control of the car), even though we *know* we are much safer on the plane. *Being* safe and *feeling* safe are two different things.

Without help learning new ways of relating to yourself and others, trauma is not "forgotten" or healed, though a person may manage it. Without experiencing yourself as safe and competent, you repeat the same reaction, the same behaviors, and probably very similar responses. Too often, we see the fear reaction and think it is a response; in other words, we think the person is choosing to act that way. My professor didn't *choose* to scream in the movie theater, any more than you would. A triggered individual hasn't *chosen* to lash out at a staff person—in that instance, it is a reaction, not a response. Unfortunately, when we confuse a reaction with a response, we might inadvertently punish the individual for his or her "behavior" or "bad choices."

Two Types of Trauma

Trauma therapists use nicknames to identify the two different kinds of trauma someone might experience: "Big T" and "little t."[31]

"Big T" traumas are the kinds of things anyone would think could cause lingering emotional problems:

- Sexual assault
- Physical assault
- Physical, sexual, or verbal abuse
- War
- Natural or manmade disasters
- Catastrophic illness
- Loss of a loved one
- Humiliation
- Chronic or severe bullying
- Captivity/deprivation and powerlessness to act on one's own behalf

According to National Core Indicators and I/DD researchers, people with intellectual disabilities are also more likely than other people to have "everyday" stresses or losses build up and become traumatic stress.[32, 33] We call this kind of trauma "little t."

"Big T" trauma is an unusual, devastating event that disrupts normal life. I sometimes joke with audiences that "little t" trauma could also be called "seventh grade." "Little t" trauma is caused by comparatively minor events that are painful or embarrassing. These probably don't affect the brain if they happen only once in a while. Let's say, though, that "little t" traumas happen to me frequently. On top of that, I don't have strategies to be successful the next time, or a support system to make myself feel loved. Over time, my brain may experience that overload of stress the same way it would during a single life-disrupting event. Some causes of "little t" traumatic stress can be:

- Living in an environment that is stressful and/or dangerous
- Chronic shortages of food, shelter, or other necessities
- Social pain and/or isolation
- Not being accepted
- Not being able to do what others do
- Moving to a new home or experiencing a significant change at home (new people in and out)
- Knowing one has a disability or is "different" from others
- Not being listened to or being misunderstood
- Failing at a task and being reminded of it
- Getting confused and overwhelmed
- Racism and other prejudices

Lieutenant Steve Click, a retired Ohio Highway Patrol officer, is a friend of mine. He now trains law enforcement and first responders about trauma, and he likes to say, "'Big T' is like being attacked by a bear. 'Little t' is like being attacked by ducks." One duck may not be a big deal, but given enough time and enough ducks, the damage starts to look the same.

POST-TRAUMATIC STRESS DISORDER[34]

I won't take a lot of space here discussing how to diagnose post-traumatic stress disorder, but I wanted you to be familiar with how that diagnosis is made. When a clinician diagnoses PTSD, we look at these four clusters of symptoms:

Hypervigilance and arousal (always on "red alert")

- Startles easily/frequently
- Shows irritability

- Has difficulty concentrating
- Has difficulty relaxing
- Has difficulty falling or staying asleep
- Needs to be near or in sight of exits, gets agitated when blocked

Avoidance
- Avoids activities, places, people, and things to keep from being reminded/"triggered" (Avoidance can ripple out and become more and more removed from obvious triggers of the original incident.)
- Can't remember important parts of the trauma
- Shows much less interest in significant activities
- Feels detached from others
- Displays a narrow range of emotions (numbness)
- Lacks a sense of future

Intrusion (having upsetting memories, thoughts, and dreams)
- Suffers from flashbacks
- Experiences nightmares
- Experiences disturbing images, thoughts, or fantasies
- Exhibits a physical response (sweating, shaking, freezing, lashing out) to internal or external triggers that resemble the event (This is very common!)

Negative alterations in cognition and mood
- Is unable to remember the event (not due to injury, medication, etc.)

- Has persistent negative beliefs about oneself or the world
- Feels persistent self-blame, guilt, or shame not realistically corresponding to the event
- Is unable to experience positive emotions

We are still learning about trauma and people with intellectual and developmental disabilities. We hope research will tell us more. In the meantime, remember that people with I/DD may not be able to verbally express the things that are bothering them, so some of these symptoms may be harder to see. We have to look for signs that a person might be upset, including nonverbal signals of distress and anxiety. Many people translate emotional distress into physical symptoms, and this can be especially true for someone with I/DD. An individual complaining of a headache or stomachache with no obvious cause might be experiencing these things because of emotional stress. This is complicated by the fact that emotional distress can go hand in hand with physical disorders. One medical handbook for working with people with I/DD lists over twenty different behaviors or movements that can be associated with mental as well as physical ailments.[35] We should monitor individuals who are nonspeaking even more closely, looking for new problems or old problems getting worse. Sometimes emotional agitation might look like:

- Rocking
- Unusual movements
- Pacing
- Stiffness
- Self-soothing
- Loss of a skill (including speech)
- Change in personality (an easygoing person becomes irritable and rigid; an engaging person seems shut-down)

- Changes in eating and sleeping patterns
- Unusual clinging or rejecting people

Nonverbal distress can be a sign of many problems besides trauma. If you notice new or increased signs like these, ask for a nurse or doctor to examine the individual.

HEALING FROM TRAUMA IS POSSIBLE— AND WE KNOW HOW IT WORKS

People heal from trauma every day. Talk therapy is a good road to start down. Language gives us the power to change ourselves. We can communicate our experiences and feel heard, redefine what we know, and find a new sense of meaning. It helps us to articulate the "unthought known,"[36] the way we see life and the way we assume things will go for us. These frameworks, these basic assumptions about the world, shape our perceptions, our sense of self, and our ability to interact with other people. Changing some of these assumptions or stories can be done with people with I/DD in many ways, such as Karyn Harvey's work with positive identity.[37] When trauma has been too early in life, too chronic or too severe, body work such as yoga, dance, qigong, or other movement-based practices might help the brain to heal "from the bottom up."

For all that we've talked about the damage that trauma can cause, it's important to remember that people do recover from it. The brain is an organ that changes with our experiences. It can be changed for the worse when those experiences are terrifying or demoralizing, overwhelming our ability to cope. But this also means our brains can heal with good experiences. Therapists recognize "post-traumatic growth" as the wisdom, self-love, healthy relationships, and calm awareness that people can have after the damage of a trauma has transformed.

Can severe traumas ever be *completely* healed? I don't know. But I've learned never to count a person out, no matter how badly hurt they've been by trauma and no matter how damaged they seem to be. Sometimes it's the most surprising people who will find ways to come back from devastating injuries. Human beings have a near-infinite ability to grow and change. Even on the last day we are alive, we have the potential to learn, to connect, to change our view about something, and to open our hearts. That is why even when people are difficult to get close to, we should never, ever stop reaching out to them.

chapter three
....

Brain Basics
(including We Don't Always Know What We Think We Know
or How I Got Everything about Your Brain Wrong)

"... an enchanted loom where millions of flashing shuttles weave
a dissolving pattern, always a meaningful pattern though
never an abiding one ..."

— Charles Sherrington, describing the brain

In this chapter, I'll talk about how the brain works. I'll also describe
how our brains change with experiences, especially trauma. But first ...

A QUICK WORD ABOUT HOW I GOT THINGS WRONG
After going to graduate school and then reading a lot of books about
the brain and attending trainings about the brain, I would usually
explain it to people like this:

The Three Brains
The three major areas of the brain are the brainstem, limbic system,
and cortex. The stack on each other from the bottom to the top, and they
evolved in that same order. An embryo develops its brain in the same
order, bottom to top, as it grows. The lower the area, the more basic the

function. The brainstem, sometimes called the "reptile brain," controls body functions. The limbic system, or "mammal brain," creates safety, memory, and emotions. The cortex, the "primate brain," does our complex thinking. It's like you have three brains in one.

Now, this description isn't totally *wrong*. But it might not be really right, either. The idea of the "three brains" became popular in the 1970s with the work of a neurologist named Paul MacLean. He came up with this model mostly from looking at the human brain and comparing it to the brains of other animals. This became the way we talked about how the brain develops and functions. This is still a popular idea, even though some brain scientists have since decided that the brain really works as a whole. All its "areas" are more like a shifting holographic map in a video game than concrete floors of a real building. But we still spent decades explaining the "three brains," with the recognizably human brain—the cortex—literally and figuratively at the top of the animal kingdom. This is a misleading image, or at least that's how Dr. Lisa Feldman Barrett, one of the world's leading neuroscientists, describes our previous views.[38] Neuroscience is changing how we think about the brain. The idea that we have the best, most advanced brains not only fits our assumptions, she points out, but it is also an *attractive* idea. More on that in a minute.

Why would we care about how we conceptualize the brain? I'm guessing no one reading this book, and certainly not the person writing it, is planning to start a side gig doing brain surgery (in your backyard, maybe, on weekends!). And I could still describe "the three brains" to you, and what you need to know for understanding trauma would be largely the same. The reason I'm telling you all this is that up until a few months ago, I was *sure* (and most neuroscientists were sure, right along with me) that "three-in-one" was an accurate way to understand the brain. And it isn't, really. I'll explain why for those people who are interested, but the point is this: Sometimes the things we *know* turn out to be wrong.

A MORE ACCURATE WAY TO THINK ABOUT THE BRAIN

A better way to talk about the brain, according to Dr. Barrett, is this: Brains mostly try to maintain our bodily resources—basically oxygen and blood sugar. Your brain takes into account all the environmental cues (otherwise known as your senses) and all the experiences you've ever had, at a speed we measure in fractions of seconds, and it prepares us for what it thinks will happen next. This way, the brain is ready to start or maintain whatever functions will keep us alive in the world. Our brain is a future-predicting machine, constantly weighing differentials to try to pick the most efficient actions to keep us going.

. . . .

Why do the brains of different animals look different?
More information for the interested

All brains start with the same genetic blueprint in their cells. The proportions of the three regions (brainstem at the bottom, limbic system in the middle, and cortex at the top) are different in reptiles, mammals, and primates because we all have different instructions for how much time an area is given to develop. Dr. Barrett uses the example of a time limit for working at a building site. In some places, you'd spend a long time building a foundation for a house because you're going to have a basement. Maybe the construction foreperson allots six weeks to dig and build that basement. In the South, where it floods, it takes only three weeks to pour a slab for the foundation, because basements aren't needed in that environment. And cells can change what they do, so the idea of dedicated regions isn't quite accurate. Cells in the midbrain may be more likely to be activated by sensory input, but the brain can reroute that so they now react to something else. For a fascinating analogy, read Dr. Barrett's description of the brain functions "networked in" together, like the global network of airports, with hubs that centralize activity. The brain's constant focus is predicting and assigning the biological resources the body needs to survive. Dogs and cats—same brain, different construction schedule. Different networking patterns = more varied functions than reptiles. Humans—same brain, different construction schedule. Different networking patterns = more functions than other mammals.

WHY THIS MATTERS: LETTING GO OF A STORY

What we "know" may not be true is good to remember—and not just when talking about the brain. It's also important when it comes to a mental illness diagnosis. When you hear a diagnosis given for someone, remember that it's a map, or maybe a better analogy is a story. If I have schizophrenia, let's say, I'm still Lara—a complicated, real person with unique characteristics. If you look at the definition of schizophrenia, some elements probably describe me perfectly and others less so. The more parts of a schizophrenia diagnosis that look like me, the better it fits me. That story will allow you to understand some things about me and predict what might help me. But I am not "schizophrenia." I'm Lara. A diagnosis of schizophrenia is a story that more or less helps you work with me. It'll give you a head start on choosing medications or the kind of therapy that might help. But schizophrenia and I are not the same thing. Schizophrenia isn't an actual person—I am. Get it?

All diagnoses are stories. Some fit a person well and are a good guide for what to expect and how to help them. Some don't fit *at all*. Many are somewhere in the middle. A diagnosis or a "story" of a broken bone is simple and predictable. It's not hard to identify the problem, and it predicts treatment really reliably. Put a cast on my arm and my bone heals straight. *The End.* In some ways, telling a story about the body can be much easier than telling a story about the mind. Complicating things is the fact that schizophrenia, from our previous example, might actually *be* a brain disease (or a gathering of diseases) that we could someday test for, like taking a blood sample and diagnosing high cholesterol. Someday the "story" of schizophrenia might be relatively easy, more like the story of a broken bone.

Stories like depression may always be tricky, because part of that story seems to involve the mind as well as the brain. With depression, it's easy to see that our habits of thought, our outlook on things, can actually impact how our brain *creates* and then *reacts to* our mood. The sadder our mood and the more pessimistic our thoughts get, the more our brain is depressed. It becomes a vicious circle, where "brain" and "mind" are *affecting each other.*[39] Changing thought habits or attitude really doesn't help schizophrenia; it's a brain disorder. Mind and body are connected, but they are not the same thing, and mind stories are, as I said, much harder to tell. Some diagnostic "stories," like defining homosexuality as a mental illness, were also considered absolutely valid and real and true. Until they weren't.

Remember, too, that these "stories" are told by fallible human beings. Some human beings are talented and thorough at their jobs, but some are not. Doctors, nurse practitioners, psychologists, and even clinical social workers (!) *can get it wrong*. Or maybe the diagnosis, the *story* they chose, fit at the time but doesn't anymore. As I said, that's one of the things about the mental health culture that can most confuse people in the I/DD world: Unlike a disability, some mental illnesses can be cured, or at least get better. A diagnosis that used to fit doesn't anymore, because the illness or problem is gone. Some diagnosticians are not good at keeping their unconscious biases out of the stories they choose. So, we can have racial or gender bias in who gets diagnosed with what. Or the science they originally based their story on changes, because that's what science does! All of this is to remind you that a diagnosis in someone's chart might be a helpful story about them, but it's not eternal, Gospel truth. It's okay to ask questions, to advocate that someone take a second look. Reasonable people can disagree, especially when someone is complicated to figure out, like many of the folks you work with. This is not to make you lose faith in mental health and related fields. We do know a lot about how people's minds and brains work, most of us try hard, and we usually do a good job. It's just to say that maybe we should all hold what we "know" lightly, because that story we're sure is true can change.

And that's not even the hardest part. The hardest part isn't when someone else gets something wrong—it's when *you* do. I had to admit (just as I was finalizing this chapter, in fact) that the way I've talked about the brain with thousands of people for more than a decade wasn't exactly wrong, but it wasn't really accurate either. A lot of neuro-scientists and science writers are going to be right there with me, a little red-faced as they change some of how they write and teach about the brain. I relied on the prevailing view of my time, so I'm not ashamed about having to admit this, really. This is how science works, as I said: We come up with an explanation that fits until a better one comes along. But I did have to swallow a little pride to write this, and that is never easy. I remarked earlier that Dr. Barrett pointed out that among all the reasons why the "three-brains-in-one" story was so accepted for so long is that of course it's appealing to us humans—we're the heroes of that story. Go, us! Best brains! And that is what can make something the toughest to let go of—*when it serves us.* When I am sure that the reason I'm having a problem with someone is *them*—their actions, their attitude, their "otherness," even their obnoxiousness (remember James?)—that is a very attractive story. *It's not my fault! What else can I possibly do?* Now, the idea that maybe I have a little something to do with this situation myself? That I might be part of the problem, after all? *Mmm ... nope. No, thank you. Much less attractive.*

So we're going to talk about the brain, what it does, and most of all, what you need to know to be able to work with someone more effectively. And I'll give you my best understanding of the current thinking, along with some resources at the end of this book if you'd like to learn more. But the most critical thing is to remember not to hold on too tightly to what you "know"—especially when it's a story that suits your feelings or your view of yourself. Be ready to be wrong, to adjust your view. Admit it when you do. Because someday, what you know might change.

We'll still talk about "this happens here" for understanding some of the basic activities in our brains.

THE CORTEX

The cortex, sometimes called "the thinking brain," is usually where we are visually imagining things, preparing for future events, speaking and writing language, and adapting our reactions to fit our environment. Controlling our impulse to yell at someone in line at the grocery store means we're responding instead of reacting in a situation where yelling isn't going to help us thrive in the group. This brain creates meaning out of symbols far away from the things they represent. Think about reading; it is *amazing*. You are looking at some squiggly marks on some pages, possibly many miles and years away from me sitting here typing them, and *you know my thoughts while I'm writing this*. All this creepy magic is possible thanks to the activity usually happening in the cortex. The cortex is busy making connections between brain cells in the early years of our life. These connections become shortcuts and superhighways for thinking and behaving. The cortex keeps "tuning and pruning" these connections between cells as we get older, depending on which connections we use a lot and which ones we don't. Some areas keep developing until we're age twenty-five or so.

Going back to the whole brain as a system: Some parts of the system have to be able to be slowed down and others sped up, depending on what we're doing. This networking *adapts* to be better at what it does a lot of. If you look at what pops up when you Google something, the sites you go to most will start to pop up first. If you stop going to those sites, they come up less frequently. The system changes itself as you use it. The human brain works in a similar way. We'll take a look at some of the basic ways this system organizes its functions, but remember: It's more like a map of flights across the world. Those flights may have regular routes, but they can be reassigned as needed. Regular routes connect things more quickly and frequently than when a route is seldom-used, but it's pure function with no fixed position in space.

THE LIMBIC SYSTEM

The limbic system is heavily involved with safety, emotion, and memory. The hippocampus is usually involved with reassembling factual information, and the amygdala is typically involved when we experience "emotional" memories. It's also the alarm center that goes off when we're threatened. It signals the body to release adrenaline, and that sets off the fight, flight, freeze, or fawn reaction when we're highly activated by the adrenaline. We shut down (collapse and dissociate) if we're overwhelmed by the threat.

The Hippocampus

This part curves up from the bottom of the limbic system and arcs around to the top, looking a little like a seahorse's tail, which is what "hippocampus" means in Greek. The hippocampus helps to organize and remember factual or "explicit" memories like information and events. If I ask you to name your fifth-grade teacher, you'd probably activate your hippocampus to pull that information. This area communicates with the brainstem, and it regulates the functions the brainstem controls, setting daily rhythms for waking and sleeping, appetite, digestion, and blood pressure. The hippocampus also communicates with the amygdala (more on that shortly). It recalls information that helps give context to what is happening. When we are calm, sensory information from the amygdala activates the hippocampus, and senses, emotions, memory, and continuous awareness all weave together seamlessly. As van der Kolk would say, the hippocampus knits incoming sensory information into a coherent, continuous story, like braiding separate strands into a single rope. This helps us calm ourselves when our environment is stressful, because the hippocampus remembers things like: "I've been through this before, and I'll be okay." Under stress, the amygdala helps inhibit the hippocampus, taking it temporarily "offline."

The Amygdala

Psychologist Louis Cozolino says, "The amygdala never forgets,"[40] and that's an easy way to remember what these regions often do: sorting through and prioritizing all the information that comes into our body through our senses. We quickly categorize any sensation: known/ unknown, safe/unsafe, pleasant/unpleasant. The most important decision our brain makes is whether something is a potential threat. Remember, your brain is always assessing the environment and trying to predict what you'll need next.

If you experienced something negative in the past, your brain instantly reacts; you yank your hand away from a glowing red burner on the stove if you've been burned before. To go back to the example I used earlier, the hippocampus is involved with how you've stored your fifth-grade teacher's name, and the amygdala might make you feel happy or tense hearing them mentioned, depending on how you felt about that teacher. Earlier, I called these sense records "emotional" memories. Once something is sorted and designated, it can trigger the powerful emotions we associate with it throughout our lives. The smell of your grandmother's house where you felt loved, the taste of the cotton candy that made you sick, the sound of a tornado siren that scared you—these may cause you to react decades after experiencing them only once, even if you were too young to have a conscious memory of it happening.

If something is unfamiliar, the brain has less information, which is why unfamiliar things make us draw back instinctively; we default to treating any new information as possibly dangerous. In other words, *things are unsafe until proven otherwise.* If something is categorized "unsafe," the brain sends a signal to activate preparing for a change in the environment. This chemical cascade sets into motion our adrenal- ized survival mode, the flight-fight-freeze-fawn reactions.

When our alarm systems are calm, they work with explicit memories to weave our experiences into the "story" of our daily lives. At the end of your day, you could tell someone about it with events in the right order and with a reasonable amount of detail, including the emotions you felt along the way. If your day is disrupted by unusual stress, the alarm function springs into action. Using Barrett's analogy of a network of airports, some airports (survival programs, body responses to adrenaline, for example) get a lot of traffic diverted to them, and the others (thinking or planning, for example) are comparatively quiet. Our usual routes for perception are thrown out of sync. This is why, under stress, we may have a hard time telling the story later with accurate details in the right order.

Imagine your boss announces there'll be a fire drill some time that day. Later, a loud fire alarm goes off. It makes the average person jump and feel slightly stressed as their brain alarm says, "Loud! Unpleasant!" It takes the brain network, talking to itself, to figure out that it's just a drill and that you can calm down. If my fear is strong (let's say I was once trapped in a burning house), my reaction might be faster and more intense. Now the safety protocol screams "FIREFIREFIREFIREFIRE!" and my brain, usually *activated* by the alarm, is overloaded. My thinking brain functions are relatively shut down as the activity is routed to survival mode. It might take me much longer, with calming sensory input (someone talking to me gently, reminding me of the drill), to start to override the panic message. Eventually I'll remember the context (the email that went out yesterday warning of the drill) and then disengage my fight/flight/freeze/fawn reaction. The brain traffic is spread out more evenly around all the airport hubs again.

The amygdala and the surrounding limbic system are also highly involved in a really important function when it comes to trauma:

bonding. A lot of the activity happening in the limbic system signals pleasure and connection to what is otherwise more of a yes/no, black/white way of experiencing the world. Sensations of physical closeness are clearly coded in our brain, and when mammals tend to or groom each other, a release of chemicals rewards that behavior. Chemically speaking, in the mammal brain, connection equals pleasure. Mammals cooperate and communicate with one another because we get such enjoyment from the feeling of being connected. We'll come back to this later on when we talk about Trauma Responsive Care.

THE BRAINSTEM

The brainstem is usually running the basic functions of the body, and it is where we see the fewest changes throughout our lives. The brainstem you're born with is pretty much the same until you die, unless your brain is subjected to extreme stress for a long time. This makes sense. You wouldn't want your brain to experiment with its plan for how you breathe; that function should be well-established by the time you're born. When the brainstem is not functioning, the brain is said to be dead. Fun fact: The guillotine (known by the name of the French Revolution-era doctor who advocated it) was considered to be a modern, humane way of killing people. Why? Because it quickly and cleanly cut the brainstem from the body.

NEURAL INTEGRATION

The brain has to move quickly and in balance for us to be thinking and feeling clearly and accurately, with our body functions running smoothly. This could be another way to say I'm in my window of tolerance: I am "neurally integrated." When trauma affects a brain over time, the network jumps too rapidly and too powerfully to those survival protocols. Thinking again about the analogy of a network of airports, imagine that instead of a blizzard rerouting a flight, all it takes is a little rain. The sky clouds over, a few raindrops fall, and suddenly all the flights are zooming to emergency routes. The person with that brain reacts faster, stays upset longer, and has a harder time thinking clearly when they're scared or angry. Noticing what we're feeling (self-awareness) and then calming ourselves down (self-regulation) gets each area of the brain working in sync at the right speeds again, with things heading in their usual directions.

WHY THIS IS IMPORTANT

When someone responds accurately to their environment versus over-reacting or underreacting, they also can be (mostly) in charge of their own mood—they can raise their low mood or soothe an agitated one. This means using some psychological strategies, like calming self-talk ("This is going to be okay") and reality testing ("Nobody is making as big a deal about this as I was afraid they would"), but all of that depends on:

- Noticing you are feeling something
- Understanding and naming what you're feeling
- Being capable of changing, or at least easing, that feeling
- Having enough emotional flexibility to change

For example, let's take the first item on the list: noticing you are feeling something. This requires internal signals in your body and brain to travel slowly and predictably enough that you can perceive them. Recognizing you are angry, thinking about the consequences of lashing out violently, and then telling yourself to calm down—all of this takes time. If the emotional part of the brain moves too fast and the analyzing, self-control parts of the brain move too slowly, you might have exploded on someone long before you even realized how angry you were. Neural integration means the activities of the brain move at the correct speed, in sync with one another, like a car in which all the moving parts connect to one another with the right timing to move the car forward. Too fast or too slow, too weak or too strong, and the car will race dangerously or lurch awkwardly.

Poor neural integration often goes along with body awareness issues. The brain, particularly the right hemisphere, takes in sensations from the limbic system and interprets them—"I feel tension in my stomach; I think I'm afraid," for example. As van der Kolk says, "You can't do what you want until you know what you're doing."[41] It's not unusual for my trauma clients to have little body awareness; they often bump into things and get injured or have trouble noticing when they're hungry or tired.

However, in order to express that feeling of fear, you have to be able to use words like "afraid." That requires—in Barrett's airplanes analogy—for hubs in the brain to harness activities all across the networks to work together to recognize and name *fear*. Inability to put words to an emotional experience—alexithymia—is often a problem for my clients. People suffering from PTSD are particularly vulnerable to this. You can't express feelings if you don't have words for them, but you can't have words for your feelings if you don't know what you feel. Since feelings are in the body, you don't know how you feel if you can't get all those networks reporting to one another—in other words, you can't feel your feelings if you can't feel your body. And that gets us all the way back to those emergency protocols, like dissociation. If I've left my body, I can't do any of this self-awareness stuff.

More Information, If You're Interested

In terms of the entire nervous system running through the body, these activities energize or slow the autonomic nervous system (ANS), made up of the sympathetic nervous system (SNS) and the parasympathetic system (PNS).

A good way to remember which system does what: Sympathetic means "with emotion." This system "goes with," or in the direction of, the emotion. Parasympathetic means "against emotion." In this case, the PNS is trying to go against, or put brakes on, the emotions.

SELF-REGULATION

Neural integration lets us understand others and respond to them. But that's only half of the equation. After we choose the "correct" response to a situation, we then have to follow through on that choice. This may mean controlling other impulses. For example, after having decided I need to keep my job, I have to tell myself to nod politely and ignore my annoying coworker instead of stomping off angrily and quitting. In order to carry out the choice I have made, I have to regulate the competing urge to act on my angry feelings. This makes self-regulation the second half of emotional regulation.

Every closed system has some way to keep itself in check. You set the thermostat at your house, and when the temperature gets too hot or too cold, the system automatically turns on the heat or the air conditioning to keep the temperature in the range you chose. As I explained earlier, neural integration allows you (the house) to know what you're feeling (the temperature). That's the first half. How you *get back into range* emotionally depends on self-regulation. How good are you at raising or lowering your mood? Can you reassure yourself when you're worried or calm yourself down when you're giddy or enraged? Many of our individuals have trouble with their emotions. They may depend on things outside of themselves (food, approval, sex, distraction, etc.) to "fix" how they are feeling, since they have a hard time regulating their emotions from the inside. People who are diagnosed with borderline personality disorder are on the far end of this spectrum; they suffer from chronic, severe emotional dysregulation, as if they live in a house where the temperatures fluctuate with no warning, swinging violently from hot to freezing with not much in between.

When I work with clients, I often start with emotional self-awareness, teaching them to ask, "What am I sensing, feeling, and thinking?" Then we practice some tools to regulate their internal state. It helps to start with calming the body, since there are more signals traveling from your body to your brain than the other way around. Working with the body versus trying to work with the brain is just faster, like driving on a four-lane highway instead of riding against that highway traffic in a bike lane.[42]

The Relaxation Response

Here's one tool I use to help my brain and body slow down. You might want to try it. Set a timer for two minutes and sit comfortably. You can sit on a cushion on the floor if that works for you, but a chair is fine too. Use as much or little support for your back as you need to sit up tall but not rigid, with your core actively holding you up. It's easier to breathe if you're not slumping, but this shouldn't feel like an effort. If it does feel effortful or your back is uncomfortable, get more support. If you're in a chair, it helps to put your feet flat on the floor if that feels okay. I like to point out to audiences that as a Petite American, my feet don't always reach the ground! Just find what helps you feel anchored and secure in your seat. You can close your eyes if that is okay for you. If that makes you uncomfortable, it's fine to just have a "soft gaze," not focusing on anything. Turn your phone over, set papers aside—basically, make your environment clear of things that distract you. Some people look at a bare tabletop, or the corner where the wall meets the ceiling.

Breathe normally, but on your exhale, imagine saying a line or phrase from a prayer, poem, or song that is meaningful or soothing to you. Don't say it out loud. "Allahu Akbar" or "The Lord is my shepherd" or "Let it be" are what I use as examples when I teach this, but it can really be anything that means something to you. I choose examples that are short, because you probably can't say a whole prayer or poem in a single outbreath. You may want to experiment a bit to find a phrase that fits comfortably with your breath. Breathe at whatever rate is natural, and just repeat your phrase to yourself when you exhale. As you do this, you may notice your heart starting to slow down and your breathing becoming more regular. You'll probably get distracted at some point, because that's what our brains do! Our brains are always looking for something to think about, and when there's not much going on, they just start popping up with random thoughts. "I'm hungry. What should I have for lunch? I should catch up on that show I started last ni—uh oh. I'm doing this wrong. I'm terrible at this!" And on and on. When this happens—and it will—see if you can notice it without getting mad at yourself and just go back to your phrase and your breath. The point is not to never get distracted. Everyone gets distracted. The point is to notice the distraction and come back.

I usually have my clients try this for about two minutes to start. If you like it and find that it helps with stress, you can keep expanding the time up to ten or twenty minutes, twice a day. This might be something you want to do before bed if falling asleep is hard for you. The Harvard doctor who developed this exercise, Herbert Benson, found out that when his patients regularly practiced the Relaxation Response, the stress levels in their bodies dropped.[43] Some of the symptoms of their chronic diseases, like diabetes and high blood pressure, got better. This was what he expected would happen. What he didn't expect was when his patients told him that when they were stressed out at work or in traffic, they could take a few breaths while saying their phrase to themselves and they would start to calm down. The more they practiced, the stronger the association was. This is not a magic spell to make you instantly serene, but remember that our brains get faster and stronger when we ask them to do a lot of something. The more you practice the Relaxation Response, the more your brain and body will connect your phrase with slowing down.

I like this exercise in particular because it's so portable. It would be great if I could interrupt a tense meeting at work and say, "Hey everybody, I'll be right back; I'm just going to go work out and then take a nap, because *you people are stressing me out*," but that probably would not go over well. What I can do in that moment is take a couple breaths, repeat my phrase to myself in my head, and start to slow down a little. Once that begins, I can use other tools to help myself manage whatever feelings I'm having. This can be a quick way to start getting myself grounded.

Brain change, healing, and learning can happen throughout our lives. This is a good thing. We learn and remember new information and practice skills until we get good at them. We mature, our reactions slow down, and we can cope with unpredictable or frustrating things in socially acceptable ways. However, this learning is bad news when it comes to trauma. Our clients who grew up with abuse may have had their brains changed by that stress. Those experiences can change the brain for the worse. Abuse can be bad for a brain, but neglect is even worse. Early, severe neglect is the most damaging thing a young human can go through; neglect starves the brain of *experience*, input from other people, sometimes to the point that critical brain areas don't develop fully or are missing completely.

Knowing our brains change, and knowing experience is one powerful way to change them, means we really need to understand *what* changes them and how to use this to help the people we support. How we perceive the world creates our experience of it. When my experiences and perceptions change, my brain changes. And when my brain changes, I change.

What You Need to Know

1. What you "know" may not stay the same, and if what you "know" happens to be a story that benefits you, it's even harder to admit when you need to change it.

2. A good diagnosis can be a helpful story, but it's not the same as the person.

3. There are areas of the brain that seem to be commonly involved with certain functions, but the brain is more of a flexible network than a rigid structure.

4. The brain is constantly trying to predict the future and assign resources to survive in the environment. It uses every experience we've ever had to guess what is about to happen.

5. It activates our survival protocols—fight-flight-freeze-fawn or dissociation and collapse—when it detects something unknown and/or dangerous.

6. If the brain guesses wrong, it sets off the survival protocols even when there's no danger. This is called being triggered.

7. This all happens much faster than we can think, and it takes time to shift the brain network back to what is actually happening.

8. The more this happens, the faster the network shifts to survival.

9. Self-awareness + self-regulation makes the difference between a brain that's operating smoothly and one that isn't.

10. Brains that have been changed by trauma can heal.

chapter four

Trauma Responsive Care: Safe, Connected, and In Control

"... Quantum physicists are not exactly sure what happens ... but they're all agreed on one thing: that reality comes into being through an interaction."

—Emily Levine

What is the quickest, most practical way to help someone when their brain shifts into a survival protocol? When someone is in fight, flight, freeze, or fawn, or when they are collapsed and dissociated? When they are reacting now to something that happened a long time ago? When they don't know who, where, or even *when* they are? How can we reach someone when fear has taken control? We can try to turn off the fire alarms in their brain and body by helping them to feel *safe, connected,* and *in control.* Trauma Responsive Care is a practical way of helping someone come back into their window of tolerance before we try to do anything else.

In order to help people reorient themselves and get back into the present, we have to get the overactive sections of their brain slowed down and the slow sections sped up. We need all parts of the brain network to be functioning in balance: Emotions are engaged, but the thinking and orienting routes are engaged, too. In this chapter,

I'll explain more about what *safe, connected,* and *in control* mean, why they have to happen in that order specifically, and offer some ideas about where you might start.

Safe

"I'd rather react to every creak I hear like it's a burglar and be wrong than miss one burglar."—Your brain

How does your brain create the feeling of "safe" in the first place? The brain sorts all the incoming information from the outside world, very quickly, and decides whether to activate your emergency alarm systems. And because the brain actually predicts what it *will* need to do, rather than thinking about what is happening in the moment, past experiences and actions that protected your safety are the blueprint for how the brain perceives and reacts in the present. A simple way to say it: Your brain will do whatever has worked in the past.

There are two kinds of safety: *Perception* of safety is when our smoothly functioning, thinking brain decides there is no threat. We can consciously act on this, like slowing down and walking calmly out of the building during a fire drill, even though the emergency siren is still going off.

When we truly *feel* safe, we know it deep in our gut. Another name for this is *neuroception*—the experience of safeness, all the way through our body. The 18th-century American preacher Jonathan Edwards talked about rationally understanding that honey is sweet versus actually tasting it and experiencing its sweetness. However logically I made myself walk slowly out of the building for the fire drill (*perception* of safety), *neuroception* is me sighing with relief, my muscles relaxing, and my heartbeat slowing when the fire alarm finally stops blaring.

If we don't feel safe in our bodies, "from the bottom up," then our actions are really survival reflexes, and our self-aware "thinking" networks will have a hard time communicating and controlling what we do.

Let's go back to an analogy for someone in survival mode. (In any of these examples, I'm assuming your individual is not in any actual danger when they are freaking out or shut-down. If there's a real threat, their reaction would be appropriate.) Take a smoke detector. If a smoke detector starts beeping in your kitchen, the first thing you do is figure out if there actually is a fire. The second thing you do, assuming there is no fire, is *turn off the beeping and reset the detector.* In a human, that means figuring out if I am in any actual danger, and then if not, convincing my "smoke detector" brain that things are safe after all.

But remember that the brain gets good at anything we ask it to do a lot. If a person's brain has been scared or triggered by trauma many, many times, their alarm system is stronger and faster than it normally would be. It also means that at the same time, those reactions create a familiar route, whereas the calm, reflecting functions have a less-traveled path to go down. So, it's probably going to take you many tries to get that person's brain and body to feel safe again. A quiet room with dim lights, fresh air outside, grass under her feet, or a blanket wrapped tightly around her—these kinds of reassuring experiences might help your individual feel secure, using as many senses as possible. When I worked for the Ohio Department of Mental Health and Addiction Services, psychiatric hospital units were making "sensory carts" for patients. These were filled with pleasant things that would trigger the senses: a fresh peppermint tea bag to smell, hot cinnamon candies to taste, brightly colored yarn to look at, a fluffy blanket or a stuffed teddy bear to hold. Administrators told me that when they used these sensory kits with their patients, they saw violent behavior, restraints, and emergency sedations all go down. The key here, I think, is remembering that the alarm system is in our *sensory networks*. We take in sounds, tastes, textures, and especially smells much faster than we can think or understand someone talking to us. If you have a close, trusting relationship with one of your individuals, the sight of your face and the sound of your voice probably start calming them long before they can sort out the meaning of what you're actually saying to them. If they are very triggered, you might have to help orient them to when and where they are, who you are, or even how old they are.

WHAT YOU NEED TO KNOW

1. Reassure your individual's senses first.
2. Try to orient them if they seem confused or dissociated. You might have to say simple things to help your individual get oriented to time, place, and self again.
3. Use directions that do this in a particular order. "Lara, it's Patrice (*orienting*). You're safe; everything's okay; you're at home *(safety)*," and so on. (We'll talk about the next step in Vicario's "safety script"[44] later.)
4. If you're helping me, then as my brain starts to answer the question "Am I safe?" with "Yes," several things happen. My parasympathetic nervous system kicks in. My brain stops sending the signal to my kidneys to pump out epinephrine (adrenaline). My breath slows and my vagus nerve starts slowing my pounding heart. My thinking brain now can get in touch with the networks that record information. For example: *The person who hurt me was Dave, and this is Patrice. Patrice is safe. I'm okay.* I start to regain the sense of time

passing and orientation. *(I'm not a little girl hiding under my bed; I'm grown up and I'm lying on the floor. I'm crying. My roommate is standing in the doorway looking worried about me.)*

Connected

In Harry Harlow's classic experiments in infant primate development, baby monkeys chose a snuggly cloth "mother" doll to cuddle up with over a cold metal "mother" doll that gave them food.

How did your talking to me help me back into my window? Given enough time, my safety protocols would have started to stand down on their own, but you sped up the process when you, my trusted, caring staff person, talked to me. Maybe you made eye contact (if I tolerate that), or maybe you put a hand on my shoulder or stood nearby if I don't want touch. When I experience this kind warmth from a person I know and feel safe with, my brain releases oxytocin and other chemicals. These neurotransmitters do many things, but in this situation, they create critical feelings: reward, pleasure, and love.

Remember we said that the brain has an on switch and an off switch for everything. The same is true for the alarm systems of the brain. The brain releases ACTH (the brain version of adrenaline) and cortisol—these are the chemicals that signal "GO!" They trigger the *flight-flight-freeze-fawn* and, eventually, *collapse* survival commands in my body. So, ACTH and cortisol are the on switch for fear. If there's an on switch, that means there's an off switch too. Dopamine, serotonin, oxytocin, and other endorphins are the chemical antagonists of ACTH and cortisol. That means they break down ACTH and cortisol in the synapses (the gaps between the nerve cells) in the brain.[45] These chemicals make the stress chemicals go away. Now we have the off switch for fear.[46] What makes our brains release these stress-destroying chemicals? Sex, food, games, gambling, laughing, drugs—all the things people find pretty fun! But one of the fastest and most powerful triggers of these pleasure chemicals is ... *love.* Human connection.[47] That snuggly feeling a kitten gets burrowing into its mother's fur triggers oxytocin, dopamine, and serotonin in both their brains. This chemical cascade motivates mammals to bond with their offspring and to stay close to pack members and mates. Seeking love, comfort, and trust with one another is right at the heart of what we recognize in ourselves as what it is to be human. When I teach audiences and students about this effect, I quote one of my favorite verses of the Bible, from the First Epistle of John: "... perfect love casteth out fear."[48] In other words, love drives fear away; love is *stronger* than fear. When we feel love, closeness, and trust, suddenly we aren't afraid anymore. Fear and love can't occupy the same space, just like ACTH and cortisol can't be in the same brain-space as dopamine, serotonin, and oxytocin. The apostle turns out to have been exactly neurologically correct. You can call it "relationship" or "rapport" if that is more comfortable, but as John McGee used to put it, we can just be direct and call it what it really is.[49]

WHAT YOU NEED TO KNOW

1. Having a close and trusting relationship already is certainly helpful, but you can help someone feel connected even if you just met them. Your gentle voice, slow words, and relaxed facial expression will be enough to get started. Think about how you would want someone to talk to you if you woke up in a hospital or were helped after a tornado hit your house.

2. We can add *connected* to the next step in that safety script. "Lara, it's Patrice. You're safe; everything's okay; you're at home. You know me. I won't leave. I won't let anyone hurt you, Lara *(connection)*."[50]

3. *Safe, connected* ... We have two of the three ingredients of the formula for Trauma Responsive Care. Now we can finish it.

In Control

"Grandma calls me *Master* Amal
because she says
I am the master of my own destiny
I am the master of my own fate
I am the master of my body, mind, and spirit"

—Ibi Zoboi, *Punching the Air*

Present, aware, interacting appropriately with the environment instead of freaking out or shutting down—that's what it means to be *in control*. This state is what we've been aiming at when your individual gets agitated, screaming, rigid with fear, or collapsed into helplessness. Of course when I say, "in control," I mean that person is in control of themselves, not suddenly promoted to "Boss of Everybody Else." Another way to think about it could simply be that a person who is in control can hear you, can make choices, can think about their actions and the consequences—whatever is normally in their range of ability. A person who is in control can take into account the feelings of others. From the brain's point of view, "in control" means all the activity of the networks in the brain are running through their organizing centers to every region of the body and working in sync with one another. Our brain assesses that the resources in the environment are safe and stable. Our body is relatively calm and we know who, where, and when we are. Your individual, when they are in control, can assess their environment accurately and feel safe (assuming, as always, that there is no actual danger present). Securely in their window of tolerance, their brain can choose what to do next. (*Should I hit this person, or should I just tell them I'm mad? What is likely to happen?*) One disclaimer: Obviously, doing all this doesn't mean the individual won't *decide* to hit that person. Things still happen, and people sometimes make bad or destructive choices. But using Trauma Responsive Care to make sure someone feels *safe, connected,* and *in control* gives them the best possible chance to be thinking and selecting among options—responding, rather than merely reacting.

Just as with *safe* and *connected*, you can help someone progress to being *in control*. Once you see a person is starting to regain some sense of themselves and seems to be slowing down (or becoming alert and present) again, you can present them with simple choices. Obviously, it helps at this stage if you have already worked out how that individual prefers to deal with feelings: a walk outside, listening to a slow, peaceful song, or organizing their baseball cards. Organizing of any kind is a good example of how to help this happen, actually. Let's take a simple deck of playing cards (this would work with an Uno deck too, which every agency and provider seem to have!):[51]

Imagine I'm just starting to calm down from being triggered. Give me the deck of cards and ask me to sort them out by color (in this example, it's a regular deck, so let's say they're black and red cards). If I need very high levels of support or can't use my hands, this might be trickier, but for the sake of the story, let's assume I can do this. Black; red; red; red; red; black. I sort the whole deck into two piles. Now ask me to find and

*sort the suits—diamonds and hearts in the red pile and clubs and spades
in the black. I can do this task without being able to read or write. Now I
have four sorted piles, one for each suit. Next, have me find the "faces" in
each pile, jack through king. If I know my numbers, then for the last step
I can put all the cards in each pile in order, ace through king.*

What do you notice about these tasks? They start out simple, with
two choices: black or red. Then they get progressively harder, with
multiple possibilities for each choice. If I go all the way to putting each
suit into numerical order, that's actually pretty complex. I'm gradually asking my thinking brain to get more engaged with each task.
This might be a nice way to help me slowly neutrally integrate—to
get the usual flights going on the most efficient, practical routes across
the globe. The networks are humming along without having to go to
emergency protocols.

What You Need to Know

1. "In control" doesn't mean someone is ordering other people
   around. It means they are in charge of their own actions.
2. To be in control of ourselves, all the parts of the brain having
   to be working together. If my brain's alarm system is blotting
   out my ability to think, I can't really choose an action. I am
   reacting instead of responding.
3. Giving me choices helps my decision-making, logical brain
   get back online. This could be a gradually more complicated
   task. You could also ask me to use logic, the next step of that
   safety script. "I won't let anyone hurt you, and that means I
   won't let you hurt anybody else, either." You can wrap up
   that script with a return to safety: "You're okay; you're safe."

Who Needs Trauma Responsive Care?

In the chapter on trauma, I talked about how widespread we believe trauma is in the I/DD community. We also know that along with being widespread, trauma is probably underreported when someone has a disability. The bigger problem is that these estimates cover only "Big T" trauma: experiences that are so out of the norm of daily life, so stressful beyond our physical capacity to cope, that even one event can cause lasting damage. But I also described "little t" traumas, the events that are not so unusual and in fact happen to everybody from time to time: feeling ignored, feeling "less than," failing at a task, having little power in day-to-day decision-making. What turns these normal human experiences into trauma is how frequently they happen and the lack of resources a person might need to change the situation. When you fail at something, you probably have ways of bouncing back— either improving at that thing so you succeed next time or finding a way around the situation so you don't have to do that thing you're not so good at. If you are a person with a developmental disability, you may not have those choices. Instead, you're confronted with things you feel you fail at day after day ... after day. We haven't even included racism, sexism, and LGBTQ+ biases and the effect *they* have on people with I/DD. Add up these stresses over decades and you may have a person whose brain is as damaged as the person with "Big T" trauma.

We already know these things. I'm repeating them here because when the I/DD field tries to estimate how many people with a developmental disability have been affected by trauma, we have no way of figuring out just how many people experience those "little t's." I've seen many versions of screening tools that identify the "Big T's" in someone's life. I've never seen an instrument that can measure how many times in a day someone feels ignored, misunderstood, devalued, or overwhelmed. Some people would argue the vast majority of people dealing with I/DD have some level of this toxic frustration and stress every day. With "Big T," we haven't gotten accurate counts yet; with "little t," there's no way to count them at all.

Given those problems, some researchers suggest more than ninety percent of people with an intellectual or developmental disability have some level of traumatic stress.[52, 53]

So, who needs Trauma Responsive Care in the I/DD community? Everybody.

Because for my money, if you say "more than ninety percent" of a group of people, you're essentially talking about everybody. I would also argue that having an I/DD makes someone vulnerable to trauma, so if they haven't experienced it yet, they're still at high risk for it in the future. If that happens, you won't necessarily know when it's happened, for all of the reasons I just went over. In the world of childhood trauma, trauma-informed care has long been a "universal precaution," and I believe Trauma Responsive Care needs to be a universal precaution in the I/DD community.

Universal Precautions: An Idea So Brilliant, It's Easy to Miss

When I worked at that runaway shelter for teens, we were constantly cleaning up cuts and scrapes from a youth's latest brawl, or dealing with a teen who came in drunk and throwing up. Our jobs included lots of blood, sweat, and ... well, worse. This was in the days of the full-blown AIDS crisis, and it was drummed into all our heads that any bodily fluids were to be handled cautiously. We were trained in universal precautions.

Universal precautions are so common now, it's easy to forget how powerful and nearly foolproof they really are (although the coronavirus has brought this lesson home to a whole new generation). The reasoning is elegantly simple: You can't tell if someone is sick just by looking at them, so the lowest cost/biggest payoff option was to treat each teen as if he or she were sick. Waiting to get a client tested for HIV, hepatitis C, or whatever would take weeks, and obviously they needed care and cleaning up *now*. But, the reasoning went, you couldn't go overboard either. I wasn't going to say, "Here, kid, take this six-week course of antivirals before I put a bandage on your cut, just in case you have something I can catch." That would have been inappropriate, dangerous, and completely impractical. Simply protecting myself was far quicker, and it was harmless to the person I was helping. It was also cheap. A few cents' worth of latex gloves and some bleach water were all I needed. Compared to the catastrophic costs of getting devastatingly (or even fatally) sick, the time and expense of treating everyone *as if* was almost zero. It's brilliant, it's easy, and it works.

In the world of I/DD, we should treat trauma as simply and effectively as we manage the risk of getting sick. Trauma Responsive Care should be a universal precaution: We should treat everyone *as if* they have some traumatic stress.

There is so much trauma we simply won't know about. If we don't weave a tighter net, we will miss most of what we're trying to catch. Assume everyone you work with has had some scary or dehumanizing experiences with other people. As a result, they have some deeply wired procedures to keep themselves safe by lashing out or by staying frozen. We may be aware of what that trauma was, or we may never know, but that's okay. With TRC universal precautions, we'll do the right things anyway. In the rare case that an individual has had no exposure to significant emotional stress, ever, this is still fine. Universal precautions really are about choosing what you want to be wrong about. If you roll the dice and "bet" that our one-out-of-a-hundred individual with no stress needs to feel *safe, connected,* and *in control,* but they are usually in their window of tolerance anyway, that's fine. They'll still benefit! After all, who *doesn't* want to feel secure, valued, and empowered? In all my years of training audiences about Trauma Responsive Care, no one has ever volunteered to feel terrified, powerless, and alone. But as I explained before, if you bet the other way—"They seem fine, probably no trauma here; they don't need TRC"—and you're wrong, you've missed something vital. Trauma Responsive Care as a universal precaution is always the smart bet. This goes for colleagues or people you supervise too. Treat each person as if they need to feel *safe, connected,* and *in control.* Act this way first, before you ask anything else of them (or of yourself, for that matter).

Who needs Trauma Responsive Care? Everyone.

chapter five

Starting with the Right Person

*"Life has no meaning. Each of us has meaning, and we bring it to life. It is a waste to be asking the question when **you** are the answer."*

—Joseph Campbell

The worst temptation most of us have with trauma is to try to "fix" the person who is dealing with it. We want to fix them because we want them to feel better. Maybe we want them to make different choices or to pull themselves out of the hole they seem to be trapped in. We also want this, sometimes, because the way that person is acting is challenging for *us*—it's weird, frightening, or upsetting. It's okay to want to not have to deal with these situations; we're human, and our motives can be selfless or selfish at any given moment. Usually, it's a bit of both. Human though it may be, this urge of ours to "fix" someone is dangerous. The most treacherous pitfall of treating people's struggles as behavior problems is that their behavior becomes all we can see, and behavioral intervention looks like the way to fix them. If we can get them to act differently, then, *Hey, look! Suddenly we're not uncomfortable anymore*. This focus on behavior can quickly blot out the *person* doing the behaving—the feelings, wants, and needs that are driving them. As I said earlier in this book, our brains and bodies are all built in pretty much the same way, and even having a significant developmental disability or a neurodiverse brain doesn't seem to change that. We are all much, much more alike than we are different. When we zero in on any one thing about a person, especially their behavior, we can forget that they're a whole, complex person. Most importantly, we forget that we often treat individuals differently than *we* want and need to be treated when we are struggling with something. I've never met any staff person, clinician, or executive who would want a committee to write up a behavior plan for them and then have a group of other people enforce it.

In fact, changing other people is impossible, even if it were a good idea (which it is not). We can offer suggestions and support, help, and hope to the people in our lives, but we cannot change them. The only thing we can change is ourselves.

Behaviorism: Revolutionary ... for Its Time

How did behavioral approaches become so dominant in so much of the I/DD field? Many of the agencies and state boards I visit as a consultant have a long history of using behavioral programs with their individuals. We started reforming how people with I/DD were treated in the 1850s, when the first modern institutions started to appear.[54] The field focused mostly on providing individuals with a decent place to live. In that context, when behavioral approaches and occupational therapies started in the 1950s, they were revolutionary tools, and they worked. Individuals could start holding jobs, and many people gained important skills. We helped ensure dignity and purpose with these advances.[55] But there are two problems with this history. The first problem is that because many of these behavioral strategies helped in many ways, it was easy to stop looking for other answers. Some areas of 20th-century mental health also focused on behavior but went on to explore feelings, relationships, and meaning—the whole person. In intellectual and developmental disabilities, though, targeting problems with behavior plans and medication are still the first, and sometimes the only, things we try. A person becomes their behavior and not much more.

Remember in the introduction when I said that, "I'll talk about why most of what you've been taught to do in those situations not only doesn't help but might be making it worse"? As a starting point, behavioral interventions make sense. Let's say sometimes a person dashes into the road. She is an immediate and real danger to herself and others. Staff want her behavior to change, and they want it to change quickly. Fair enough. So, her staff and maybe a behavior specialist or psychologist try to figure out how to get her to stop doing this. They ask themselves what comes right before the person's running episodes; maybe when she gets too little sleep the night before and she's frustrated or sensory-overloaded, she's more prone to run. Looking more closely, they see she tends to pace and mutter right before she takes off. And finally, as the weeks go by, someone points out that she really loves dancing to club music, and that if her staff can catch her pacing and muttering early enough and engage her in dancing with them, they can head off her bolting.

Now there's a behavior plan. It's humane, detailed, and reasonable to use. So what could be the problem? Well, there isn't one so far as the plan goes. The problem comes in when the person's team understands her just enough to change what she's doing. That may well mean they're putting a bandage on a deeper issue that never gets resolved.

My business partner and I have consulted with a lot of providers and state agencies across the country, and we've seen behavior plans that are a great starting point—a good way to get quick improvement in someone's care, and the beginning of staff getting to know that person. Unfortunately, we've also seen many behavior plans that were the beginning *and* the end; as long as an individual's behavior changes the way people want, it goes no further. There's not a compelling reason to understand what they're feeling, to build a relationship, or to try to provide the interactions or the experiences they need to heal. When I worked in children's mental health, we reminded ourselves of the same potential trap in our field by repeating this saying: "Sometimes parents just want us to make their children good; our job is to make them well."

I think I get how this stopping-at-the-surface happens, with the best of intentions. Remember the conditions in which so many I/DD (and mental health) services are provided. Too many staff people and managers are underpaid, hastily trained, and poorly supported, sometimes working from instructions that are not completely explained (or incorrectly designed in the first place). English may be a second language. Staff may have a lot to do and not enough time in which to do it, with people who act in ways that can be strange, exasperating, or dangerous. Given all that, simply getting me to stay in the house and not dart out into the road suddenly seems like an understandable place for my care to land. But it isn't enough, for two reasons.

Number one: What happens when the plan doesn't work? If the emphasis is on getting someone to do what they're "supposed to do" (and that definition can veer quickly from their staying safe to their compliance and docility so the day runs smoothly), then you can easily feel justified in focusing *only* on the person's behavior. Then it's a short step to doing just about anything to get that behavior in line. It probably starts with ignoring the individual. (That's a subtle distinction from what is probably in their plan already: Ignore their *behavior*. How exactly you are supposed to do this without ignoring *the person* is a fine needle to thread). From there we move to punishment: isolating, scolding, shaming, and more extreme measures. When all else fails: meds. I will never say medication doesn't have its place; sometimes the medicine that treats mental illness and emotional distress saves lives. But in the I/DD population, there can be problems[56] with doses that are too high, or several medicines within the same "class" (say, multiple antidepressants at the same time), or a new medication that's been added without any old ones taken away.[57, 58] All this means the population we serve is at risk of being seriously overmedicated. It's hard to avoid the idea that sometimes medication is used primarily to keep someone's behavior under control for the comfort or convenience of others. That's chemical restraint. And it's abhorrent.

This, of course, brings us to physical restraint. Physical restraint and other aversive behavioral techniques can cause trauma or make it worse.[59] If restraints were used perfectly, with absolutely every measure taken first, and applied only when absolutely necessary, that would be one thing. We know that's not the case.[60, 61]

I supervised staff in some comparable situations with young people with emotional disturbances and mental illness. I know that when staff get burned out, frustrated, and angry, they usually demand more consequences for the people they are trying to work with. What they sometimes really mean when they say, "We need more consequences!" is they want more ways to control behavior. If we used all the tools at our disposal in our field (restraint, isolation, medication), we'd have the power to control whatever our individuals do. But we might also end up overmedicating, disempowering, and essentially imprisoning people in the name of caring for them. And that is too much power for one human being to have over another.[62] These worst-case examples don't happen all the time—maybe not even most of the time. But making behavior not just the first but the *only* priority sets the stage for all this to play out.

All of that is just Reason Number One that behavior should not be our focus; now we move on to Reason Number Two.

Trauma is not about behavior. Disordered, disorganized, bizarre-looking, or dangerous behavior can be the result of trauma, but trauma itself is an injury someone has suffered, not a decision to annoy others. As it usually happens to the people in our care, that injury was caused by other human beings. It erodes our individuals' ability to tolerate people. At its worst, trauma robs people of the ability to tolerate themselves. Addressing behavior, *and only behavior*, misses the core of the damage trauma causes: the damage to the relationship with others and with the self. Missing that damaged core means we miss the opportunity to heal it. Having a relationship with another human being who is consistent, caring, and supportive, someone who wants their individual to feel safe and in control so she can act from her best self—*this* is that person's best chance for getting better. If the focus is on directing, shaping, and controlling someone instead of joining with them, it's just too easy to miss the point completely. It doesn't help our individuals find the awareness and self-determination, the positive identities, and the authentic lives we want them to have. "Behavior management systems that focus on controlling behaviors from the outside will never build deep values and internal control."[63]

Behavioral strategies have their place. They can be powerful ways to teach someone, and for some people, they're a potent inroad to communicating. But behavior strategies are limited, and using them as both the road and the destination misses some problems and causes others. Behavioral systems make, as the saying goes, "good servants and bad masters." Treating people with traumatic wounds that are invisible to us, as many of our clients have, can only spell trouble if we rely on purely behavioral approaches.[64] A level system, for example, is a great teaching tool, especially if you want to teach someone about ... level systems. It may motivate some people, but others will use it as just another hoop to jump through and it still won't change anything about how they relate to other people or themselves. The great humanist psychiatrist Irvin Yalom said it best: It is the relationship that heals.[65]

I learned all this in graduate school when I was studying clinical social work, and I have taught the same thing to my students over the years. The truth is, though, that I learned this hard lesson mostly from the failures in my own life. When I am being grouchy or unreasonable, there is a part of me that can hear myself snapping and being childish. It has taken a lot of practice and hard work, but I can usually change my behavior (in this case, talking meanly or overreacting) with some sort of calming self-talk. ("This is okay; it's not a big deal; you're fine" is what it usually sounds like in my head.) Until I feel relatively okay, my behavior doesn't change much. For a long time, I was convinced that if the other person changed what they were doing, then I could change what I was doing, but certainly not before. I would decide, *They have to act better first!* So, I would put a lot of angry effort into getting that other person to change how they were acting so that *I* could act appropriately. I argued with them, explaining just exactly how wrong they were. Sooner or later, I'd lose my temper when, unsurprisingly, trying to control that other person didn't work. Finally, after many years of this, I realized that I *have* to change me and that I can't ever change someone else, no matter how hard I try. I can tell someone how their behavior is affecting me ("I don't like it when you yell"), but I can't insist that they quiet down so *I* can stop yelling. I have to focus on what I am doing and how this does or doesn't create the situation I want. Matching someone's anger by screaming at them to stop being angry probably won't bring peace—just more screaming. There's no way around this truth. And the fastest way for me to change what I'm doing is to start with me, on the inside. When I feel upset, I'm usually worried something bad is going to happen or that I won't get something I want. Sometimes I'm embarrassed because I think I've done something wrong or said something that makes me look dumb. Maybe my ego is threatened and I feel defensive. My brain is answering the question "Is Lara safe?" with "Nope!" And I get more and more upset. When I can look inside myself and kindly deal with my feelings (like that self-talk I mentioned before), I start to relax. My brain starts answering "Is Lara safe?" with "Yes" or at least "Getting there." And suddenly, changing what I'm doing seems possible again.

As I start to feel safe, it helps if I can remember that the person across from me probably doesn't think I embarrassed myself. Sometimes I remind myself that things will usually work out somehow. In other words, I begin to settle down. Then, changing my tone becomes surprisingly easy, and I can back up, apologize, or at least communicate clearly and skillfully. Sometimes my changing does seem to help the other person change what they are doing too, and that's a plus, but it is not the goal.

I sometimes talk with my clients about their "inner weather," a shorthand term for their sensations, feelings, and thoughts. We always work with that as the primary goal, rather than changing or fixing the people in that person's life. You are only in charge of the weather inside of you—you can't change somebody else's weather for them.

The Golden Square:
Attunement-Attachment-Attention-Adjustment

How do we learn to do this? Where are we starting from in our own childhoods? I've created the Golden Square of attunement, attachment, attention, and adjustment to illustrate the answers. This image is one way to think about the processes that shape how we react to things, and then notice and work with those processes so we can react to things appropriately and intentionally.

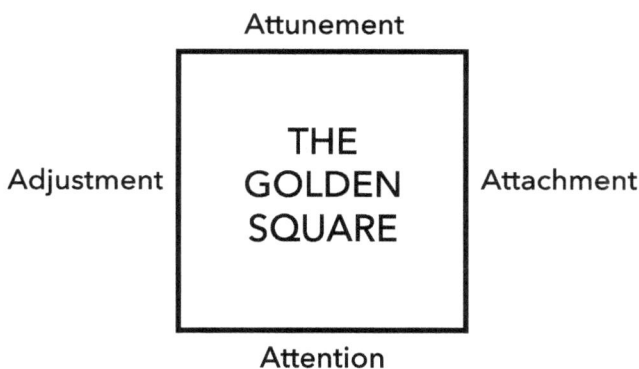

Attunement

Adjustment	THE GOLDEN SQUARE	**Attachment**

Attention

Attunement: The First Side of the Square

Attuning means matching, or getting "in tune" with, someone else on a deep emotional level. There are some people who seem to have that magical knack for settling people down, just by talking quietly with them. Sometimes their simply being in the room brings the temperature down. These people probably don't have actual magic powers, or spells that only they know, to soothe that difficult person. The "magic" they have is, among other things, good attunement skills. I knew a man who worked in a facility for youths who had committed sexual offenses. He told me the staff there had a nickname for those magical people who could de-escalate situations with the often-volatile young people in their program: "solid objects." The common wisdom there was that some staff people could maintain their composure no matter how upset a young person was, and this was deeply reassuring to the youth. They could attune—get on the young person's emotional wavelength and gently bring their own peaceful emotions into the young person's emotional range. Then the young person would gradually lower their emotional energy to match the emotional energy of the staff. This is such an unconscious process that the young people were probably unaware of what was happening; they just knew they felt reassured and heard.

We learn attunement early. When a baby cries, our natural human instinct is to pick up that baby, smile at it, and talk to it to soothe it. Every time this happens, that person is giving the baby signals with his or her facial expression, voice, body tension, and possibly even smell. The message is this: "Everything is okay. You are loved and safe." This message is different from what's happening in the baby's brain and body. The baby's brain and body are agitated and upset, overwhelmed by the feelings that made the baby cry in the first place. Bessel van der Kolk describes it this way: "We start off *being* our wetness, hunger, satiation, and sleepiness ... incomprehensible sounds and images press in on our pristine nervous system."[66] After a while, soothing tones and gentle movements help the baby gradually calm down until her brain and body activity match those of the person holding her.

The baby goes through this process over and over: Baby feels upset; caregiver calms and soothes; baby feels calm and relaxes. This sequence "programs" the baby's brain and nervous system, setting that internal thermostat I mentioned earlier. This process of gradually matching brain states between baby and caregiver is *attunement*.

For most of us, our caregivers were consistent and calm enough that our baby brain got used to what it feels like to go from upset to relaxed. Not only did our brain start to "wire in" the pattern (upset-calming down-calm), but we also learned something important: When we're upset, we'll be helped and taken care of until we feel better. We learned that the world is, for the most part, a safe and welcoming place. Most caregivers learn how to keep *themselves* calm, even when a baby is screaming and fussy. They have their own needs taken care of so they can pay attention to the needs of the baby. Their environment is healthy and predictable enough that there is routine and safety every day, so they will probably do what English pediatrician D.W. Winnicott famously described as a good-enough[67] job of caregiving. Here, "good enough" doesn't mean, "Meh, okay, I guess." It also doesn't mean "perfect." It means "sufficient." Babies don't need perfection; if the caregiver can be present and calm most of the time, that'll do. This baby will get enough of what she needs. The caregivers will create that pattern over and over for her, and her brain and body will learn safety and self-soothing. If the caregivers have a hard time doing this because they have to pay constant attention to surviving, or the environment is so chaotic they spend most of their energy just trying to get through the day, or they are distracted by their own depression, anxiety, mental illness, addiction, or violence, it's hard to make things soothing and safe enough, often enough, to program that little baby brain for emotional equilibrium.

What we learn to expect from caregivers becomes what we unconsciously expect from the world. It governs how much we allow ourselves to get close to others, and we call that pattern of interaction *attachment.*[68]

Attachment: The Second Side of the Square
There are three basic attachment styles:

Securely attached. This is how most of us experience the world when we are very young. We handle new things with some curiosity, we trust that we and other people are basically good, and we feel relaxed enough when we are around people we love and trust that we can let people get close to us.

Insecurely attached. This style has two branches: anxious and avoidant. If we *didn't* get enough repetitions of calm soothing when we were babies, or our environment was chaotic or stressful, we may have become **anxiously** attached. As adults, we worry we won't get what we need from other people, so we either grab onto anyone who seems like they will be nice to us, or we push people away before they can make our worst fears come true and fail to love or protect us. Surprisingly, a lot of the time we do both. Someone starts to make us feel loved and safe, the way we wanted to feel when we were babies, and we rush into intimacy or trust with them. At the same time, the feelings they give us are so precious that we worry they will be taken away from us. This worry makes us angry and resentful (anger is usually the top layer of hurt or fear). We can't stand how worried we are about losing those good feelings. We may fear we'll be dependent and helpless, powerless without the person who gives us the feelings we crave. So, we get rid of the fear and resentment by pushing that person away or denying the feelings that, deep down, we want and need. Anxiously attached adults can go from one to the other state (clingy to angry), confusing themselves and the people around them. It can be hard to have long-term romantic or friendly relationships with someone who has this pattern of lurching back and forth, from craving to pushing away.

Some people spend most of their time at the angry, resentful end of that arc, and they protect themselves by always staying distant—sometimes to the point that they see other people as objects or obstacles, not as fully human. This is the **avoidant** branch of the insecure style. Manipulators, adults who have difficulty recognizing or caring about the feelings of others, and even sociopaths may have this style of attachment.

Disorganized. The last kind of attachment is disorganized. This pattern is the rarest, and some people describe it as a combination of anxious and avoidant. Babies who attached in a disorganized way have highly fearful, unpredictable reactions to people. Adults with this style may seem erratic, deeply distrustful of others, volatile, and sometimes show behaviors that can look bizarre. The extreme reactions in people diagnosed with Borderline Personality Disorder, for example, may be the result of a disorganized attachment style.

Attention (Self-awareness): The Third Side of the Square

Remember earlier I talked about the fact that emotions are in the body. This has a lot to do with the vagus nerve, that "wandering" nerve (named from the same word root as "vagabond") that travels from our head down through our core. This nerve acts as the brake on our powerful heart.

We think we have an emotion in our head and then our body responds (we get scared and our heart starts pounding). But consider if it actually works the other way: Your heart starts pounding, this information travels up the vagus nerve to your brain, and your brain says, "Oh! I must be scared!" Trauma therapists often get their clients to pay attention to what sensations they are having in their body in order to learn to recognize and work with emotion. People who spend a lot of time outside their window of tolerance often feel either agitated or shut down but rarely present and calm.

They experience their emotions as a tornado that sweeps them away from their thinking self, and even their awareness of where, when, or who they are. So, noticing their emotions, starting with their body "from the bottom up" as Bruce Perry would say, helps them pull the tornado apart and start to name each feeling. "I'm freaking out" or "I feel nothing" is too big and too vague to get your hands on. "I feel scared, defensive, and worried"—each one of those separate emotions is something you can deal with in turn.

So the third side of the square is paying attention to what your feelings feel like for you and then learning to name them. We'll come back to this idea in the next chapter when we talk about the CALMER Skills. Being able to tell at any given moment what you are feeling helps ground you in the middle of that Golden Square.

Adjustment (Self-regulation): The Fourth Side of the Square

I talked about self-regulation earlier. "Adjusting" means that ongoing dance between ourselves and our environment. We take in information about what is around us (our senses); we react in a way that is mapped out, in part, by our early experiences and the people around us when we were infants (our attachment style). We communicate back to the outside world with confidence, curiosity, and interest or avoidance, fear, and aggression. The world around us does—or doesn't—change based on what we put out there. The dance goes back and forth, endlessly. Sometimes I imagine it's like waves washing up on a beach. The shape of the wave changes as it hits the sand, but it also slightly changes the shape of the shore each time, on and on, back and forth. The ability to adjust, to change what we are telling ourselves on the inside and make decisions about how we act in order to better fit the outside world, makes the difference between a healthy, positive dance and a trapped, destructive one. When it plays out as an unchanging cycle, it can mean the difference between a life that is fulfilling and productive versus one that is wasted on anger, isolation, and misunderstanding. To adjust to the environment (and to communicate what we want and need so it can adjust to us), we need those two sides, attention and adjustment, or self-awareness and self-regulation.

BUILDING THE GOLDEN SQUARE

In our work, adjustment also means using the skills we have and the knowledge of the person we're with, then watching and shifting to help meet their needs. I like using a hug or reassuring touch when someone is upset. Attention (self-awareness) means knowing that *I* like that, but that's a personal, inside feeling or preference of mine, not a universal truth. Some people can't tolerate touch, especially when they're upset. Adjustment (self-regulation) means resisting the urge to hug someone just because it makes *me* feel better, with the excuse that it's "for the other person." Adjusting might mean using my observation and skill to see that the person I'm working with actually needs more physical space from me, not less. The skill is in backing off without backing away, staying in communication to help them feel safe, connected, and in control without imposing my own needs and wishes on the situation.

Here's another way to think about this. Education expert Becky Bailey talks about how teachers of young children do a lot of the emotional regulating *for* their preschoolers, because self-awareness and self-regulation can be thought of as two selves—one self watches and observes what the other self is feeling.[69] Preschoolers haven't developed that yet. For many adults, the "watching self" can do the soothing that calms down the "feeling self." Children typically don't have their inner voice until about age seven. They only have the feelings. So, Bailey says, the teacher is the other, watching self that can do the calming for the child. Sometimes the individual we are working with has those two selves inside them, the watching self and the feeling self, and they just need support and time to get that regulating system, the conversation between the two selves, back online. When someone talks kindly to me even when I'm being cranky and controlling, my "watching self" can step in more quickly. If both of us are yelling, it can take much longer before my second self has a chance to chime in and calm my "feeling self" down.

Some people we support don't have that "watching self." Maybe they will develop it or maybe not. Either way, we are sometimes the "watching self" for them, the voice that can report kindly on what we see, giving an encouraging message to the person who is very much in their "feeling self." We might say, "I can see you're having a really tough day; you look angry and upset. Let's figure out together what will help." Our inner weather can help regulate theirs; we can't expect controlling their behavior to regulate their state, just like someone trying to control me when I'm grouchy would only send me into immediate, intense anger. Our goal is working with the "state" of the other person, not controlling them or changing their behavior. Bailey notes that when we focus on behavior, in reality our goal (whether we say it or not) is usually just stopping the behavior.

To sum up, we need to work with the right person first, and that person is ourselves. With others, we need to have the right goal: focus first on the inside (feelings), not the outside (behavior). We could put "attention" and "adjusting" (self-awareness and self-regulation) together into what Bailey calls the "skill of composure." This means being the person you want the other person to be.[70] I think of composure as presenting a self that is in control of feelings—acknowledging them but not letting them run the show. A self that is behaving in ways that support the feelings of others and adjusting appropriately to the environment.

Working with our emotions, our reactions, and our thoughts gives us space, a little breathing room to slow down. When we slow down, just for a fraction of a second, we can choose how we want to respond. Doing this is hard. Practicing doing this helps us to be present, to be thoughtful—to help *ourselves* feel safe, connected, and in control. When we can do that, we can help the person in front of us feel that way too, now that we've started with the right person.

In the next chapter, "The CALMER Skills," is a step-by-step guide to getting ourselves grounded so we're standing with our feet planted inside that Golden Square of emotional balance.

chapter six

The CALMER Skills

"Do you have the patience to wait until your mud settles, and the water is clear?"

—Lao Tse

People who have been traumatized can be exquisitely sensitive to other people's energy. Being able to read someone's moods may have helped to keep them safe—it might even be how they survived. Trauma can turn survivors into human X-ray machines; the tiniest shift in the expression on someone's face or a hint of tension in a voice can set them off. Some of the people we work with in I/DD can be even more perceptive about mood, especially if they are good at receptive communication (hearing) but limited in expressive communication (talking). If you're faking something, they'll know, probably before you do. This all means that paying attention to how we feel and working with our own "weather" is not an extra thing we can add if and when we feel like it. It's the key to every interaction we have with the people we serve. For managers, it's the key to anything you do with your staff. We have to be mindful of the Golden Square: recognizing how we observe and match the feelings of others (attunement), knowing how we tend to experience other people (attachment), noticing how we are feeling in the moment (attention), and understanding how we can shift that (adjustment). Remembering when and how to do that can be hard, especially when we are stressed or in the presence of someone who is dysregulated. This is why Trauma Responsive Care relies on the CALMER Skills.

AM I IN MY SQUARE OR NOT? OR
WHEN SHOULD I USE THE CALMER SKILLS?

How do you know where you are? Standing in the center of your square, grounded and present, can feel expansive and open. Looking out in four directions, you can see a wide range of choices. You can see the emotions of the person opposite you, but they aren't overwhelming you or freaking you out. You can think and feel at the same time. You can modify what you're doing to get the best outcome for your situation.

What does it feel like when you're *not* in your square? You feel cornered, or like you're in a tunnel and you can see only one outcome. You're worried about how you look. You might feel small, terrified, or furious. You might be checked out, spacey, or numb. These reactions aren't in your conscious control, but how you work with them is. As we saw in the chapter about the brain, the part of your brain trying to keep you safe is much older and faster than the thinking network that notices and identifies internal emotional states. If that "smoke detector" thinks you're under too much stress, it'll knock you into hyper- or hypo-arousal *long before* you realize what's happened. The best we can do is to notice the train we're on after it's pulled out of the station and headed down the tracks. Once we've figured out where we've gone, we need to have a map to get back. The CALMER Skills can be your map.

As we work with ourselves, we'll start with three commandments about what feelings are and how they work.

THE THREE COMMANDMENTS OF FEELINGS

The first step in understanding feelings is to recognize when they are happening. In order to do this, we have to be connected to our bodies. Think of expressions like "my heart sank" to describe feeling disappointed or "my stomach is in knots" when you are nervous. Our language reflects what we intuitively know—that our emotions are rooted in our body. If you notice two people talking in a foreign language and you can see them clearly but you can't understand them, you probably can still get the vibe between them. This is because you can see their expressions and how they are gesturing or moving; you see their emotional states reflected in their bodies and faces. In your own life, you might find that your emotions get away from you easily—you act on them before you are aware of them. Do your cheeks burn when you're embarrassed? Maybe your voice quavers when you're scared or your fists clench when you're angry. Learning the cues from your body will help slow that process.

Here's a way to practice this: Stop reading this page and ask yourself what cues you notice in your body at this moment. It may help to do a body scan. Start by getting quiet and then noticing sensations, from your feet to your head. What's going on in the core of your body? See what you might observe, like a tight or nauseated stomach, tense muscles, or fast breathing. Do you notice cool, hot, or prickling skin? Are you flushed or clammy? Are your hands clenched? Are your feet tapping nervously? As you practice tuning into your body awareness, you'll start to see what happens when you feel each of these basic emotions:

- Anger
- Sadness
- Fear
- Happiness
- Embarrassment/shame

The first commandment of feelings is that feelings are in the body.

In my private practice, I work mostly with trauma and grief. I often see people who are feeling profound sadness and loss. If I could somehow offer them the chance to not have known the person they loved, so they could avoid the pain of losing them, every single one of my clients would turn me down. They'd rather have had that person in their life, even knowing the anguish that was to come. Love and the pain we feel when we lose it are inseparable. Both are important. Emotions tell us what we treasure, where we've been, who we are. So we have to value emotions, even the difficult ones. Being cut off from our feelings, feeling nothing, feels worse than feeling everything.

Sometimes I describe emotion as energy, like electricity. Is electricity good or bad? Obviously, it's neither—it's just a force. If it's powering cities and running computers, electricity is "good." If it's a bolt of lightning setting fire to my house, then it's "bad." But these are our interpretations of the results, not the force itself. Emotions are the same. Anger is the perfect example of this. Many of us have had negative, even damaging experiences of anger, either our own or someone else's. But anger, like all other emotions, truly is *value-neutral*. It can powerfully motivate for good, if someone gets angry enough to fight injustice or insist on change. Anger might be what moves an individual to stand up for herself. Still, if I have had negative experiences with anger in my own life, it might be deeply uncomfortable for me when an individual I'm working with is angry. Subtly (or not so subtly) I might discourage or discount their emotion. But even if we could do it, removing anger from our individuals' lives would do them a disservice. Anger is neutral and anger is a part of us.

If emotion reflects our human experience, then limiting someone's emotions limits their humanness. We have to decide that we recognize, value, and encourage *all* emotions, in ourselves and in others. We can't decide to acknowledge only the feelings we like.

The second commandment of feelings is that all feelings are value-neutral.

The next thing to keep in mind is that no matter how much we love or hate how we're feeling at any given moment, that feeling will end and a new one will take its place. Emotions are energetic states in the body and brain, and energy *moves*. Emotions constantly change, sometimes subtly and sometimes dramatically, but they never stay the same for long. Even in the depths of the greatest pain, if they can just sit and watch their feelings, my clients notice that their emotion gets a little lighter or changes to something else. They'll stop crying for a minute, smile, and tell me a funny story about the person they loved, and we'll laugh. In a while, that too will turn to something else. In the midst of depression or anxiety, our feelings may feel agonizingly unending, but even then, if we look closely enough, we'll see them morph into something different, like clouds changing shape. Many of the ways we treat anxiety, for example, involve teaching people to observe their feelings, no matter how uncomfortable, until they notice the anxiety start to fade. Sooner or later, it always does. This fact in and of itself makes their anxiety less scary. If we accept that feelings are neutral, we also have to understand that they never last forever.

The third commandment of feelings is that feelings are temporary.

The CALMER Skills

Now that we've laid the groundwork for understanding feelings, let's go back to that idea of a map to follow when you realize you're not planted in your Golden Square anymore.

Working with feelings and mindfulness has been discussed by many different writers. As I was learning about this years ago, Daniel Siegel's book *The Mindful Brain*[71] was an important foundation for me. His COAL model helped me build the CALMER Skills, and Siegel's readers will recognize some of those elements adapted here.

When we feel extremely stressed and anxious, it can be hard to gather ourselves enough to focus enough to work with our feelings and thoughts. If that's how things are feeling for you, take a break and get some air or maybe a few sips of water to help your body regulate a little. Remember the Relaxation Response from chapter three? If you liked that exercise, you might want to start with it here.

Now you're ready.

C: Check In

We begin by checking in with ourselves. What am I sensing, feeling, and thinking right now, at this moment? Asking yourself that question is "checking in." The more often you do it, the easier it will be to tell what's going on inside you. If you experience anxiety or depression or you have traumatic experiences of your own, you might be nervous about allowing yourself to feel much. Skilled therapy can help with all of those problems. You deserve to be able to fully feel and to truly inhabit your own life.

A: Accept

Knowing how you feel doesn't help much unless you then accept whatever that feeling is. This can be easy to say and hard to do. We have been told from childhood what feelings are acceptable and which aren't, which ones make men "strong" or "weak" and which ones make women "bitchy" or "doormats." But remember the second commandment: *All feelings are value-neutral.* All feelings have their own validity. If you're feeling something, you're feeling it.

This doesn't mean your feelings are always accurate. If someone hurts your feelings, you feel hurt, and that's not to be questioned. That doesn't mean the person meant to hurt you or even that you interpreted the situation right. Maybe you didn't hear them correctly. You might be wrong about the whole thing—but you aren't wrong about your feelings. We don't always need to act on our feelings; in fact, it's usually a good idea to wait before acting. But if we don't accept how we're feeling as an internal fact, then we try to ignore or deny that feeling. That might work for a while, and if it's a fleeting moment of exasperation or whatever, then ignoring might be a good strategy to let it dissipate. But when feelings are strong, or come back again and again, acting like they're not happening doesn't help. In fact, one of two things usually happens: Either the feeling grows until it gets away from us and then comes out in unexpected, uncontrolled ways, or we cut ourselves off completely from our emotions.

That's the serious problem with chronically ignoring our emotions. When you don't let yourself feel something, you end up numbing yourself from all other feelings as well. You can't select what you do and don't feel. You have to shut it all down. Given enough time, this becomes how you move through the world: numb and disconnected.

We have to accept every feeling we have; nothing should be rejected. One way to work on this is to decide to try to treat each feeling with compassion. Again, this doesn't mean you have to *believe* that feeling. You can honor a feeling without assuming it reflects ultimate reality.

Imagine you're comforting a child who's crying because he had a nightmare about a monster under his bed. How would you talk to that child? You probably wouldn't yell at him or ignore him or pretend you couldn't hear him. You also probably wouldn't run screaming from his room, terrified of the monster. You would comfort the child and treat his emotions kindly and respectfully, without believing there was an actual monster. You wouldn't buy into his interpretation of reality, but you would be accepting and compassionate with his feeling. This brings us to the next step in CALMER ...

L: Loving-Kindness

You can read this phrase two ways. The first way is a traditional meditation practice and mindset that goes back to early Hinduism and Buddhism.

The second way is simpler and just means, "Be nice to yourself." Being lovingly kind to yourself in the moment might mean you take a few seconds to remind yourself you're doing your best, or that you succeeded at some small part of this challenging situation. It might mean taking care of your body—stopping in a tense moment to step outside, get a breath of fresh air, or take a drink of water. This can actually help us re-regulate our brains and stop our emotions from driving our actions. The example I always use in trainings is low blood sugar. I have it, and if I forget to eat, I get woozy, clumsy, and irritable. If I notice that my blood sugar's low, I have a choice: I can get mad at myself for letting it happen (which increases my cortisol and adrenaline, driving my blood sugar *even lower*), or I can just ... you know, eat something. It doesn't have to be a big deal, and caring for my needs works much better than yelling at myself about it. "Lovingly Kind" just means talking kindly to yourself and maybe doing something nice or comforting for yourself. At the least, breathing and drinking a glass of water are always a simple place to start.

M: Mindful

"Mindfulness" means a lot of things to a lot of people these days—it's become kind of a buzzword in countless articles and even commercials. Here it just means, "Notice what is and isn't happening around you *right now*." When I worked at that crisis shelter for teens, I saw a lot of on-the-edge situations blow up or settle down depending on how the people in charge reacted. In particular, if we had to call the police to deal with something, I saw how powerfully their approach could affect the outcome. Officers who talked calmly, listened carefully, and were slow to react usually helped resolve the situation peacefully. If the police came in loud and aggressive, ordering people around and not listening, ready to react to the smallest hint of trouble, I knew for sure that things were going to get worse and somebody was leaving in handcuffs. We were lucky; most of the officers who were dispatched to us knew our program, and they often did a great job with our emotionally volatile teens (and sometimes our teens' angry, intoxicated parents). A smaller number of them went to the opposite extreme and made situations much worse than they started.

When you've seen a potentially explosive situation blow up, often it's because a staff person, family member, law enforcement officer, or someone else in power overreacted. After all the hubbub dies down and the incident reports are written, when you ask that person why they reacted the way they did, their answer often ends up being some version of "Well, I was worried that (whatever bad thing) was *about to happen*" (emphasis mine). Not that it *was* happening, but that it was *about to happen*. Those are two different things. It's tricky to tell the difference sometimes, and to be fair to the people in these examples (including the police), sometimes things get dangerous quickly and it can be best to take precautions. Let's use the example of me as a client who runs. If you see me pacing and muttering near an exit, then positioning yourself by the door in case I make a break for it just makes good sense. Running across the room and tackling me because you were "worried about what was about to happen" does not. That would be too much; you'd be overreacting. So in CALMER, the "Mindful" step means taking a second to ask yourself, "What is *actually happening right now* (versus what I'm afraid *might* happen)?" Then do something if it's needed. If it's not needed, then give things a minute to slow down on their own. Don't let your fear or frustration decide for you what you should do.

E: Express

In our work, it's easy to feel frustrated, powerless, confused, overwhelmed—name an emotion, you've probably felt it. Our work is stressful, and we might be connecting with individuals who spend a lot of time dysregulated and upset. If you are a naturally empathetic person, you feel what they feel, and when our individuals feel sad, angry, lonely, or frustrated, it's hard not to pick up and carry those emotions ourselves. In a stressful situation, it might be crucially important to share what's going on with you, even just for a few moments of support and venting. When our emotions are validated (not "do whatever you feel," but "whatever you feel is okay"), it can let off some steam. We become regulated and in control of ourselves, and once again the thinking self is back in the driver's seat. When I am flustered and upset, I simply cannot think calmly enough to make good decisions.

In several agencies where I've worked, staff shifts would start with a brief meeting about the clients, and we would include a quick check-in about how we ourselves were feeling that day. Sometimes this was a formality; other times, staff came in with their own stresses or worries, and this was a chance for them to unload their feelings in a safe environment and set them aside so they could focus on the shift ahead. It helped staff to feel closer to one another and built camaraderie.

In our experiences as consultants, many of the providers my business partner and I work with take their employees' stress seriously. They try to make sure their staff have a safe place to vent and feel heard. If your agency isn't providing regular chances to express your thoughts and feelings, lobby for that. However, even if you do have those opportunities at work, it may not be enough, especially if you work with very traumatized, reactive, dysregulated people. We know from decades of research that people who are in direct contact with others who are distressed build up their own distress. Just by showing up at work, you are at some risk for emotional wear and tear. Add to this the fact that you have a life, with your own stresses, pressures, and history.

In the trainings my consulting firm does, I emphasize that each one of us needs to think about where we get support in our personal lives. You may be good at letting people around you know you need their help, but many of us helpers are actually pretty terrible at that. I suspect it comes along with being a caregiver—we like the idea of helping others, but we're not so crazy about the idea of needing help ourselves. You also might be in a situation where it's enough of a challenge just getting through your week. I've been lucky enough to talk to a lot of staff people, managers, and clinicians across the country. So many people had highly responsible jobs; complex, challenging individuals to work with; *and* stressful personal situations, such as single parenting, family members with special needs, or households to support. It can seem counterintuitive, if not ridiculous, in the middle of all that to think about taking time to talk to someone and get your own emotional first aid. Like so much of what I've been talking about here, what seems like frosting ("I'll get to it if I can") is truly the center of the cake (which I guess is just more cake). It's a cliché and you've seen it before, but it's a good one because it's true: If you're on a plane and there's trouble, you have to put your own oxygen mask on first. The flight crew warns you of this because if something happens to the cabin pressure and the emergency masks come down, your instinct is to take care of the person next to you, especially if it's a child or someone vulnerable. You need to fight that urge. You *have* to put your mask on first, because you're no good to anyone if you pass out. Then *nobody's* breathing.

So, think of it this way: If you need to vent after a tough shift, if you need to talk about the pressures at home or the stresses of your personal history, you're putting an oxygen mask on. Then you'll be there for the people you care for. Talk to a friend after a shift, talk to your manager after a tough week, talk to your pastor or clergyperson, talk to a therapist, or write in a journal. Many providers offer access to Employee Assistance Program counselors or other outlets. Find something that works for you, *and then do it*. The people in your life need you to be breathing.

R: Respond

Now, after all this, you're ready to respond! It may seem impossible to do all of this instead of just jumping in. This is a lesson I learned when I was on call for emergencies in the crisis shelter and later when I worked in a partial hospitalization program: When situations are moving fast, you have to slow down.

You have time to do this.

You can think of this as really just a longer version of the point I made earlier in this chapter. When things are (metaphorically) on fire, our instinct is to run around even faster, putting the flames out. What I learned, after doing it the wrong way many times and exhausting myself without being terribly effective, is that stopping to gather everybody, calm down, and make a plan really didn't take much time. Almost anything, no matter how stressed or crazy, can wait a minute while you take a timeout to get together, prioritize which problems need to be handled first, and decide who will do what. (The exception, of course, is an actual fire—in which case, get everyone out first and plan second.) Even in a fire, if you watch the professionals work, you'll see they move quickly but not frantically to assess what's happening, and they'll take the few seconds they need to coordinate with their leader. *Then* they spring into action. *When situations are moving at their fastest, you have to slow down.*

Going through all these steps can take a long time or a very short time. You can spend hours going through this protocol, and if you're decompressing after a particularly upsetting shift, that might be exactly what you need to do. You can also do each one of these things in a matter of seconds. It might not be the most thorough process ever, but you can ...

- Take a couple of breaths.
- Ask yourself what you're feeling (Check In).
- Accept whatever the answer is (Accept).
- Say or do something supportive for yourself (Loving-Kindness).
- Notice what is and isn't happening around you *right now* (Mindful).

- Talk with someone, now or later (Express).
- Finally, take appropriate action (Respond).

... all in 120 seconds or less. Take another moment or two and help someone else through these steps, if you can. Now you—and your team, if you have others around you—can decide what to do without being panicked or shut-down. You can assess things accurately without over- or underreacting, and you can take care of yourself, at least enough to get through the shift and then come back to it in more depth later.

Special note to managers and supervisors: In the I/DD world, there aren't as many opportunities to check in as a team and do this in the typical service provider setting or group home. I still encourage you to create a quick, easy routine for staff to talk a little about how they are doing and to practice using CALMER. They can do this with the other person they are relieving on duty, in a shared logbook, or at least at your regular staff meetings.

There should also be an outlet for emergencies, a trusted manager or supervisor who can give flustered staff a moment to vent before jumping into problem-solving. In all but the direst crises, there's a moment to talk, listen, and regroup as a team before plunging back into the situation (see Mindful, above). During a chaotic day, this pause to talk about how they are feeling can seem irrelevant to you. It depends on whether you think staff responding appropriately and skillfully is irrelevant. *No, it's not?* Of course it isn't. You want staff to be effective. Going through this process with them can be a key to getting the results you want. You need your staff to be grounded and thinking clearly. Giving them a familiar routine to offload feelings regularly, and a quick vent for stress when things get hectic, is the goalpost—not the sidelines—of what you are trying to accomplish.

chapter seven

The Main Points in This Book

Mental illness and intellectual/developmental disabilities can happen in the same person. Many people in the I/DD field understand this better than people in the mental health world.

Trauma is a common mental illness (or injury) and is commonly missed or misunderstood. The people we serve with I/DD are no exception, and they may be more vulnerable in some ways (both to having trauma and to having it go unrecognized).

Trauma is about how someone is reliving their toxic stress now. It's not in the past, even if the original event is, and being pressured to "let it go" won't help.

Traumas can be a single life-changing event ("Big T") or countless small stressors ("little t"). They can add up to the same thing over time.

We all have our typical range of functioning in our brains and nervous systems, our "window of tolerance." When confronted with a threat, we go into a hyperaroused state (fight-flight-freeze-fawn) or a hypoaroused state (collapsed or dissociated) to survive. This happens much faster than our conscious brains can think.

These protocols are built in at the earliest layers of our brains. They are not symptoms or pathologies.

Behavioral approaches can be helpful, but we have to use more than that or we miss what's crucial about trauma, and about people. They should be tools, not the whole toolbox.

The brain is a unified force made up of countless, changing paths and functions, all bent to a single purpose: predicting and adjusting to make sure our bodies have the resources they need in any given situation. A brain that has experienced toxic stress will predict danger even when it's not present.

Ideas (about the brain and everything else) change.

Trauma, especially when it's early, intense, or repeated, can affect everything about a person. As Bruce Perry would say, the state becomes a trait. This is how someone's trauma can make us fundamentally misunderstand them.

Trauma is about being unsafe and out of control. Trauma Responsive Care is making sure the person in front of us feels safe, connected, and in control before we ask anything else of them.

Because we can't know who has experienced trauma, and we know many of our individuals have, Trauma Responsive Care is

a universal precaution. Everyone should be treated this way, all the time.

It's tempting to want to fix or change people when their survival protocols are getting in their (or other people's) way. But that's the wrong approach.

The person we work with first is *ourselves*. We need to be aware and ready to work with our *own* reactions and protocols.

The Golden Square (attunement, attachment, attention, and adjustment) is a metaphor for understanding how we developed our emotional patterns and how to work with them in the moment.

The basic emotions are happiness, anger, sadness, fear, and shame. Bonus: Anger is usually a secondary emotion, a reaction to hurt or fear.

The Three Commandments of Feelings:
   Feelings are in the body.
   Feelings are value-neutral.
   Feelings are temporary.

The CALMER Skills can get us into a reasonably grounded state when dealing with situations at work. They may also help in our own lives. The CALMER Skills are:
   Check In
   Accept

Loving-Kindness
Mindful
Express
Respond

These calm, grounded interactions, repeated over a long time, create the conditions for brain change and healing in our individuals. Skilled, self-aware relationships are the way through.

All this makes you "the way through" for the people who need you.

The Way Through

"The only way out is the way through."

—an old saying

At the beginning of each semester, I'd write that quote on the board for my conflict resolution class. It's always nice to start something with a quote. It gets people's attention, and usually someone has said something you haven't thought of before—or at least they've said it in a jazzier way. I chose this quote every year because conflict is pretty uncomfortable for most of us, and we were going to spend several months together trying to notice that uncomfortableness but hang in anyway to resolve disputes. Most of my students didn't go on to become mediators or negotiators, but their jobs were going to include managing lots *and lots* of conflict: fistfights between residents, heated battles in a family session, tense negotiations in agency meetings.

Working through a conflict can feel messy and scary. I think this is because the outcome of a conflict is uncertain, and we humans generally hate uncertainty. I'd argue that even so, that discomfort is usually better than what we're stuck with when we avoid a conflict. Avoiding the mess almost always means the problem sticks around, and it typically only gets worse with time. So in this class, we'd study skills and practice roleplays for navigating conflict effectively, but most of all students had to learn to notice and manage their own discomfort. We'd come back to that quote again and again, reminding ourselves that the only way to really get past the uncomfortable situation was to deal with it.

Making ourselves available to someone who is in pain can be pretty tough. We have to try to remember that the individual (who maybe is currently trying their best to haul off and punch us) is actually *afraid* and is worthy of our compassion and presence. Working out how to reach that shut-down staff person who seems to be nothing but negative and resistant is, honestly, a big pain in the butt. It all takes time none of us feels we have. But my argument to you is this: It's worth it to go through to the other side, even if you have to take the long way to get there.

In another course, about integrating Eastern and Western treatment methods, one of the texts I used was a smart, insightful book about Buddhist approaches to therapy called *Going to Pieces Without Falling Apart*, by Mark Epstein.[72] If you're interested in using mindfulness and nonattachment while helping people, you might want to check it out; Epstein is engaging and wise. One passage I would read aloud to the class was about an experience the author had with his in-laws as the family tried to figure out how to clear a path at a vacation house. They wanted a quick way to get from the house down to the beach, through a dense patch of trees and bramble. One option was to bulldoze through the woods and lay down a straight, concrete walk. Fortunately, he writes, they decided instead to take the time and trouble to make the walkway wind and twist through the huge, old trees, rocks, and brush rather than cutting it all down. It made construction more complicated, and the project took more time to complete, but they ended up with a pretty, curving stroll through the woods—and they still got to the beach. *It took longer, but it was worth it.*

I respond to this story, I think, because when working with my clients in therapy, I've always pictured us as being in a dark forest together. We walk slowly along; they tell me their story and I learn about their life, their character, their strengths—and their wounds. Some of their stories are harrowing, and it can feel dangerous and scary to be on this journey with them. We try some things; when they don't work, I feel like I ran smack into a boulder. Sometimes a question I think will tell me a lot ends up going nowhere, or the client gets distracted and now we're stuck in some thorny briar patch of a tangent. If therapy goes on for a while without results, I have moments when I worry that I'm lost and I'm leading us in circles. But if I can stay patient and trust the path, something *does* work; a confusing experience suddenly makes sense, some pain diminishes. In my head, the trees fall away and we're in a sunny, open meadow, at least for the moment. Given time and patience, we find a way out of the forest and life gets better for my client. They can feel, and connect, and grow. They reclaim themselves as a full person, here in the present day, no longer stuck in the past.

Now, that path-through-the-forest image might sound really far away from the daily reality of your job, slogging through a long shift, sitting through a meeting with an angry family member, or tiredly stretching your budget for the hundredth time to keep services running. As someone who has walked with human beings carrying unthinkable pain—and watched them heal as they found their way— let me tell you something with perfect confidence: *You are doing more than you think.* Even if your individual never makes it into a therapist's office, your willingness to learn about trauma, to try to respond in a new way, to give them a chance to experience humans as safe, caring, and predictable, helps to keep them on that path to wholeness. It takes courage to notice and work with your own sometimes-uncomfortable feelings so you can be present with theirs. It takes dedication to give someone a chance to learn to trust you and themselves. That's how you help people to feel regulated, balanced, grounded, and able to predict their world. And with enough days feeling enough of those things, people start to heal.

Every time you give someone that chance, you help them find their way. It may take a long, long time. The path might never be smooth, straight concrete. But it is the only way out, and many of you reading this right now, no matter how discouraged you feel, are *the right person, in the right place, to walk with them.*

I'm a trauma therapist, and I believe passionately in the power of skilled psychotherapy to help people recover from even the worst wounds life inflicts. My dad is a pharmacist, and as I like to say to audiences, *I am a big fan of drugs.* This usually gets a laugh, but it's also true. The right medicine, in the right dose, can help someone with their everyday anxiety or bouts of depression. Sometimes medicine accomplishes the nearly miraculous. We have drugs that can save people from the isolation, terror, and misery that severe mental illness can be. We don't have a medication specifically to treat the profound damage caused by serious trauma, but a good, sensitive prescriber can help to manage mood, agitation, insomnia, and other symptoms so life can be bearable enough to work on healing.

Therapy, meds, extra treatment with art, music, and drama, and other interventions—I wish every individual with I/DD and trauma had access to all of these things. We still don't have enough of those resources ... yet. Maybe that will change. Strange to say, that doesn't worry me too much. This is what I said in the introduction:

"Understanding and working differently with trauma, in everyday interactions, really can be a key to healing it." While we're waiting for the day that mental health treatment is widely available and easy for anyone to find, our individuals still have the best chance there is at healing. They have that, because they have *you*. If I had to choose between all those tools and treatments and medications or you, I would pick you every time. The daily interactions that feel loving and validating ... those repetitions of routine, support, and encouragement that slowly, slowly help someone feel that the world can be safe and they can be powerful in it? Those relationships are the most powerful medicine for traumatic wounds—and you bring that medicine to work with you every day. No drug, no intervention, no behavior strategy at our disposal can do better than that. Our brains exist to make sure we have the resources to survive. They try their best to predict what is coming next. Your interactions teach your individuals that "what comes next" might be okay. For humans, "okay" means warmth, connection, safety, the power to act, and the power to move. Your individuals' brains are built, in other words, to heal and thrive on what you can provide every day. Gradually, their brains can change. When their brains change, even a little, everything starts to change.

You can put a different ending on stories of horror and neglect. You can help people live their true lives, as their authentic selves. There is no way to calculate the value of that for the people we serve, those who are trying to find their way out of a dark woods into the light.

There is a Buddhist saying that "Compassion is the best healer." I am profoundly grateful that there are people like you, with the compassion and the commitment to do your work, unglamorous and frustrating as it is. I hope you'll bring that same compassion to yourself, as well—this can be a long, hard trip through the forest. Thank you, on behalf of all the people who cannot thank you themselves. Thank you for being willing to learn, for being willing to try, for showing up for the people we serve. Thank you for staying with them, all the way through.

....

chapter eight

Questions

"Whatever is rejected from the self appears in the world as an event."

—Carl Jung

Some of these questions might be useful for you. Any question that doesn't seem to apply to you, or that asks things that you don't want to answer, just skip.

PART ONE: FEELING BASICS

Anger

What do you notice (from your feet to your head) in your body when you are angry? *Example: upset stomach, sweaty palms, shaky voice, red face*

_____

_____

_____

_____

What thoughts do you notice? *Example: This shouldn't be happening to me! This had better stop!*

_____

_____

_____

_____

Can you allow yourself to feel this feeling?

_____

_____

_____

_____

What helps you feel better physically when you notice this feeling?

_____

_____

_____

_____

What changes do you notice in your body, emotions, and thoughts when this feeling changes?

_____

_____

_____

_____

Fear

What do you notice (from your feet to your head) in your body when you feel:

i. Scared? *Example: butterflies in stomach, shaking hands, tight throat*

ii. Hurt/sad? *Example: "pit" in stomach, tight chest, watery eyes*

_____

_____

_____

_____

What thoughts do you notice when you feel scared? *Example: I can't handle this; this person/situation is going to cause me damage or trouble.*

_____

_____

_____

_____

Can you allow yourself to feel this feeling?

_____

_____

_____

_____

What changes do you notice in your body, emotions, and thoughts when this feeling changes?

_____

_____

_____

_____

Hurt (Sadness)
What thoughts do you notice when you feel sad/hurt? *Example: I can't believe this person is doing this to me. They're so mean.*

_____

_____

_____

_____

Can you allow yourself to feel this feeling?

_____

_____

_____

_____

What changes do you notice in your body, emotions, and thoughts when this feeling changes?

_____

_____

_____

_____

Embarrassment/Shame

What do you notice (from your feet to your head) when you feel embarrassed or ashamed? *Example: Sick to your stomach, racing heart, flushed face*

_____

_____

_____

_____

What thoughts do you notice when you feel embarrassed or ashamed? *Example: I look like I can't handle this; this person/situation is making me look bad.*

_____

_____

_____

_____

Can you allow yourself to feel this feeling?

_____

_____

_____

_____

What changes do you notice in your body, emotions, and thoughts when this feeling changes?

_____

_____

_____

_____

Relaxed/Calm

What do you notice (from your feet to your head) in your body when you feel relaxed and calm? *Example: Feet are "on the floor," chest is open, face is smiling*

_____

_____

_____

_____

What thoughts do you notice when you feel relaxed and calm? *Example: This is going fine; I like this person/situation; I'm good at this.*

_____

_____

_____

_____

Can you allow yourself to feel this feeling?

_____

_____

_____

_____

What do you notice in your body, emotions, and thoughts when this feeling changes?

_____

_____

_____

_____

Part Two: Triggers

What are things that can trigger feeling angry for you?

a)

b)

c)

What are things that can trigger feeling scared for you?

a)

b)

c)

What are things that can trigger feeling hurt/sad for you?

a)

b)

c)

What are things that can trigger feeling relaxed and calm for you?

a)

b)

c)

PART THREE: THE GOLDEN SQUARE

Attunement

I know someone is attuning to my feelings when they ...

_____

_____

_____

_____

I am aware of the feelings of others when I ...

_____

_____

_____

_____

A time that I was successful reading the feelings of someone else was ...

_____

_____

_____

_____

Attachment

When I was little, I knew the adults around me were in their window of tolerance when they acted like this/said these things:

_____
_____
_____
_____

When I was little, I knew the adults around me were in their hyper-aroused, fight/flight/freeze/fawn state when they acted like this/said these things:

_____
_____
_____
_____

When I was little, I knew the adults around me were in their collapsed/dissociated state when they acted like this/said these things:

_____
_____
_____
_____

When I was little, the adults around me handled their feelings by:
a) Talking out their feelings
b) Acting out their feelings
c) Shutting down their feelings

When I was little, I learned from the adults around me that conflict is usually:
a) A good chance to learn about others and myself
b) A bad, shameful thing to be avoided
c) A dangerous thing to be afraid of

I think the adults taking care of me were:

  a) Mostly good at attuning to babies and soothing them

  b) Sometimes good and sometimes not so good at that

  c) Often not great at attuning

I often feel in my heart that the world is:

  a) Basically safe

  b) Unpredictable

  c) Cold

I often feel in my heart that the people in my life:

  a) Will take care of my feelings and try not to hurt me

  b) Sometimes try to control me by how much I need them

  c) Should be used before they can hurt me

Attention

When I am in my engagement zone/window of tolerance, I notice these sensations/feelings/thoughts happening with me:

_____

_____

_____

_____

When I am in the fight/flight/freeze/fawn state, I notice these things happening with me:

_____

_____

_____

_____

When I am in the collapsed state, I notice these things happening with me:

_____

_____

_____

_____

Adjustment
I know I am changing what I'm doing when I:

_____

_____

_____

_____

A time I successfully adjusted to a situation with someone was when:

_____

_____

_____

_____

PART FOUR: SELF-EXPRESSION
How skillful do you feel at expressing yourself when you feel:

Angry

1	2	3	4	5
No skills		Some skills		Lots of skills

Scared

1	2	3	4	5
No skills		Some skills		Lots of skills

Hurt/Sad

1	2	3	4	5
No skills		Some skills		Lots of skills

Embarrassed/Ashamed

1	2	3	4	5
No skills		Some skills		Lots of skills

Relaxed/Calm

1	2	3	4	5
No skills		Some skills		Lots of skills

In which areas would you like to gain more skills?

_____

_____

_____

_____

PART FIVE: CHARACTER STRENGTHS AND VALUES

Character Strengths

What are your highest scores for character strengths? (See the Values In Action questionnaire at valuesinaction.com.)

a)

b)

c)

What do you notice in your body, emotions, and thoughts when you feel you are using your character strengths?

_____

_____

_____

_____

Which character strengths do you most want to use around other people?

_____

_____

_____

_____

Values
What values do you think are most important to live by?

_____

_____

_____

_____

What do you notice in your body, emotions, and thoughts when you feel you aren't living up to them?

_____

_____

_____

_____

What do you notice in your body, emotions, and thoughts when you feel someone else isn't living up to them?

_____

_____

_____

_____

acknowledgments

Many of the people listed below helped me with this book. Any errors are mine, not theirs.

I would never have written this book if I hadn't started working at the Ohio Department of Developmental Disabilities (DODD) and the Ohio Department of Mental Health and Addiction Services (then ODMH). And *that* would not have happened if my friend and colleague Kevin Aldridge, running policy at DODD at the time, hadn't called me with a crazy suggestion to apply to manage a joint project between those agencies. It was scary and exciting, and it opened up a chance for me to do two things I really love: *weaving together disparate disciplines* and *helping people do something useful.* I worked with fascinating people and learned a lot. Since then came several more adventures, like starting a small-but-mighty policy think tank and finally embarking on consulting and training on our own. (Kevin would like me to mention at this point that our consulting firm is **Aldridge Palay Consulting,** and yes, please feel free to contact us.) This business, along with my private practice, gives me meaningful work every day and I am profoundly lucky to get to do it. Kevin talked with me about the shape of this book and how to reach the audience I wanted it to have.

Thank you, Kevin.

The National Association for the Dually Diagnosed (NADD) has been a resource for thousands of individuals, professionals, and families. I'm proud to have spoken at their conferences, met their amazing staff and members, and now written a book for their press. I would like to specifically and gratefully acknowledge the enthusiasm and vision of CEO Jeanne Farr. She championed this book and this topic.

Thank you, NADD and Jeanne.

Writers often talk about how helpful a talented editor can be. I found that to be true working with Jennifer Scroggins—not just in catching my mistakes (of which there were many) but also by helping me shape and refine sections of this book. Plus, she laughs at my jokes. This book has also been made better by the beautiful designs of Mark Sullivan.

Thank you, Jennifer and Mark.

I have gotten to work with dedicated, talented people all over the country (and beyond), and I never stop learning from them. A few of them need to be mentioned by name here, but trust me, there are many more. Dr. Karyn Harvey, Juanita St. Croix, and Mary Vicario lent me their time, encouragement, and kind permission to quote from their work. I'm proud to know them.

Thank you, Karyn, Juanita, and Mary.

I also would not have been able to do this without the chance to teach at Ohio State University's College of Social Work as a lecturer in the MSW program. My decade there was instrumental in helping me to hone and clarify my thoughts. I appreciate every student who showed interest in the topics we covered: Trauma, grief, integrated Eastern and Western approaches, conflict, and clinical diagnosis. I loved every minute of it—well, grading not so much, but the rest of it was a joy.

Thank you, OSU College of Social Work students, faculty, and administration.

My husband, Darren Thompson, has supported my career, emotionally and tangibly, every day. His belief and encouragement are irreplaceable for me. He did all this while co-raising our family and blazing his own distinguished professional path as an artist and educator. Our sons, Liam Thompson and Aidan Thompson, are smart, compassionate young men I'm lucky to have in my life. All three of them kindly read or discussed this manuscript and gave me ideas to improve it.

Thanks; I love you.

My family—Myron Palay, Margaret Arrowsmith, Xan Palay, and Patrick Palay—are unfailingly encouraging. Margaret Arrowsmith is also a therapist, and she has been a role model for me since the day I started as a clinician.

Thanks, everybody!

• • •

Finally, I dedicate this book to the memories of two people: Jim Lantz and Liz Palay.

Jim Lantz was one of my graduate thesis advisors and quite simply my favorite professor *ever*—simultaneously entertaining and instructive, at times moody and a big pain. Beneath his cranky Appalachian exterior, he was compassionate, insightful, and wise. He put me on the road to understanding trauma from an academic, clinical, and human perspective. He was a powerful influence on the generations of students he taught.

This book is for my professor, with gratitude.

My mother, Liz Palay, was a professional historian of science and technology *and* a master's-level hospice social worker in the course of her varied career. She was wickedly smart, deeply driven, extremely funny, and once for a bet she wrote a murder mystery novel in a week. Mom won the bet—and it was a pretty good mystery too.

This book is for my mother, with love.

index

ADHD. *See* attention deficit hyperactivity disorder
adrenaline, 20, 39, 54
anxiety, 2, 3
attachment styles, 75-77
attention deficit hyperactivity disorder (ADHD), 3,4
ACTH, 55, 56
alexithymia, 44
arousal, brain, 13-19
    adrenalized, sympathetic state, 14-15
    collapse, dissociation, 15-16, 20
    hyperarousal, 14
    hypoarousal, 14
    social "engagement zone," 13-14
    "window of tolerance," 13-14, 17-18, 20, 43
autonomic nervous system (ANS), 45

Barrett, Lisa Feldman, 32, 33, 34, 37, 41, 44
Bailey, Becky, 79-80
behavior management, 6
behavioral disorder, 2
behaviorism
    medication in, 69-70
    physical restraint in, 69
    shortcomings, 68-69, 98
    strategies, 70-71
Benson, Herbert, 48. *See also* Relaxation Response
Big T vs. little t trauma. *See under* trauma
bipolar disorder, 3, 4
borderline personality disorder, 3, 4
brain
    amygdala, 38, 40-42
    arousal. *See under* arousal, brain
    brainstem, 31, 33, 42
    changing understanding of, 31-33, 36, 98
    cortex, 33, 37-38
    development of, 31, 32, 33
    effect of neglect on, 49
    hippocampus, 38-39
    limbic system, 33, 38-42, 44
    midbrain, 34
    models of, 31-33, 36
    neural integration, 42-43, 45
    purpose of, 98
    "reptile brain," 32
    regions of, 31-32, 55, 98
bullying, 24

CALMER Skills, ix, xviii, xvii
    Accept, 88-90, 99
    Check In, 88, 99
    Express, 92-94, 100
    Loving-Kindness, 90-91, 100
    Mindful, 91-92, 100
    Respond, 94-96, 100
    when to use, 84
Click, Steve, 25
COAL model, 88
collapse, 55. *See also under* arousal, brain
composure, skill of, 80
connection, need for, 55-57
control, need for, 57-59
cortex. *See under* brain
cortisol, 12-13, 20, 55
Cozolino, Louis, 39

depression, 3
    resolution in, 8
    thought habits and, 35
developmental disabilities
    duration, 8
    as mask for other issues, 5
    source, 8

diagnosis
  bias in, 5-6, 36, 60
  as story, 35, 49
diagnostic overshadowing, 5-6
direct services professionals (DSPs),
  xv-xvi
dissociation, 16-17, 44. *See also*
  hypoarousal
Dissociative Identity Disorder, 16
dopamine, 55
dual diagnosis
  as misdiagnosis of trauma, 3
  recognition of, 97
  treatment duration, 8-9

Edwards, Jonathan, 52
emotions. *See* feelings
endorphins, 55, 56
epinephrine, 54
Epstein, Mark, 102

fawning, 15. *See also* fight, flight, freeze,
  or fawn.
fear
  ACTH and, 55
  brain reactions, 23
  collapse and, 16
  cortisol and, 55
  expression of, 44
  PTSD and, 44
  in trauma, xvii
  vs. love, 55, 56
feelings
  basic, 85-86, 99
  physicality of, 85-86
  temporary nature of, 87
  "three commandments" of, 85-87, 99
  value-neutral, 86-87, 89
fight, flight, freeze, or fawn, 15, 17, 20,
  39, 41, 49, 51, 55

*Going to Pieces Without Falling Apart:
  A Buddhist Perspective on Wholeness*
  (Epstein), 102

Golden Square, xvii, 73, 99
  adjustment, xvii, 73, 78-79
  attachment, xvii, 73, 75-77
  attention, xvii, 73, 77-78
  attunement, xvii, 73-75
  building, 79

Harlow, Harry, 55
Harvey, Karyn, 28
hippocampus. *See under* brain
hypervigilance, 13. *See also* under Post-
  Traumatic Stress Disorder
hyperarousal, 14
hypoarousal, 14

intellectual or development disorder (I/
  DD)
  indicators of mental illness in, 27, 97
  nonverbal expressions in persons
  with, 27-28
  See also dual diagnosis; development
  disorder
intermittent explosive disorder, 3

Janet, Pierre, 11, 18

learned helplessness, 16
limbic system, 13, 33, 38-42, 44
little t trauma. *See under* trauma: Big T
  vs. little t

MacClean, Paul, 32
McGee, John, 56
medication, 2, 6
  as behavior control, 6, 7, 69
  off-label use, 6
  overuse, 69-70
  trauma and, 104
mental health treatment
  culture, 8
  caregivers' self-perception, 7, 99
  finite nature of, 36
mood disorders, 2
  misdiagnosis, 4-5

See also specific disorders
Multiple Personality Disorder, 16

National Core Indicators, 2
neglect, effect on brain, 49
neural integration. *See under* brain
neuroception, 52
networks
  neural, 41, 42-43, 44, 49, 50, 51, 53, 54
  sensory, 54

obsessive-compulsive disorder (OCD), 3
OCD. *See* obsessive-compulsive disorder
oppositional defiant disorder, 3
orienting, 54
overfocusing, 13
oxytocin, 55, 56

parasympathetic nervous system (PNS), 45, 54
Perry, Bruce, 17, 98
personality disorders
  misdiagnosis, 4-5
  See also specific disorders
polyvagal theory, 13
Porges, Steven, 13
positive identity, 28
post-traumatic growth, 28
Post-Traumatic Stress Disorder (PTSD), 4, 21
  avoidance in, 26
  diagnosis of, 3-4
  effect on mood and cognition, 26-27, 44
  hypervigilance, 25-26
  intrusion, 26
PTSD. *See* Post-Traumatic Stress Disorder

Reiss, Steven, 5
Relaxation Response, 46-48

restraint, 69

schizoaffective disorder, 3
schizophrenia, 3, 4, 8, 34-35
safety
  need for, 52-55
  perceived, 52
  true, 52. *See also* neuroception
  See also safety script
safety script, 54, 59
self-regulation, 45-46, 78-79, 80
sensory carts, 53-54
serotonin, 55, 56
sexual assault
  and misdiagnosis of trauma, 3
  of persons with disability, 2
  as source of trauma, 24
  underreporting, 2
Siegel, Daniel, 88
sympathetic nervous system (SNS), 45

Tenex, 6
therapy, 6, 103
trauma-informed care, xviii
Trauma Responsive Care (TRC), xviii
  defined, 51
  elements of, 52-59, 98
  need for, 60-61
  reacting vs. responding, 22-23
  as universal precaution, 62-63, 98-99
trauma
  age and, 21, 98
  appearance as other disorders, 4
  behavior and, 70
  Big T vs. little t, 24-25, 60, 97
  causes, 24-25
  coping strategies, 21
  development of, 12, 20-21, 24
  hormone response, 12-13
  in persons with disability, 2-3, 27, 60
  interpersonal, 19
  misdiagnosis, 3, 4
  persistence, 12, 21, 97
  prevalence, 2, 60, 97

recovery, 9, 28-29
single-event, 9, 97
as "social brain" injury, 19
triggers, 18-20, 21, 50
understanding, 8
untreated, effects of, 18
See also Trauma Responsive Care
(TRC)

universal precautions, 61-63. *See also
under* Trauma Responsive Care
(TRC)

vagus nerve, 13, 54, 77
van der Kolk, Bessel, 11, 15-16, 18, 21,
39, 44
Viagra, 6

window of tolerance, 51, 55, 97. *See also
under* arousal, brain

Yalom, Irvin, 71

Source Material and Recommended Reading

(in alphabetical order)

7½ Lessons About the Brain by Lisa Feldman Barrett

The Body Keeps the Score: Brain, Mind and Body in the Healing of Trauma by Bessel van der Kolk

The Brain that Changes Itself by Norman Doidge

Conscious Discipline by Becky Bailey

Gentle Teaching by John McGee

Going to Pieces Without Falling Apart: A Buddhist Perspective on Wholeness by Mark Epstein

The Identification and Treatment of Trauma in Individuals with Developmental Disabilities by Sharon McGilvery

The Mindful Brain by Daniel Siegel

The Neuroscience of Psychotherapy: Healing the Emotional Brain by Louis Cozolino

The Pocket Guide to Polyvagal Theory by Steven Porges

The Polyvagal Theory in Therapy: Engaging the Rhythm of Regulation by Deb Dana

Psychotherapy for Individuals with Intellectual Disability, Robert Fletcher, ed.

Trauma and Memory by Peter Levine

Trauma and Recovery by Judith Herman

Trauma Practice: Tools for Stabilization and Recovery by Karyn Harvey

Trauma Responsive Care: A Training Manual by Lara Palay and Kevin Aldridge

Who Am I?: 16 Basic Desires That Motivate Our Actions, Define Our Personalities by Steven Reiss

Endnotes

1. I've altered identifying details of this story and others in this book to protect privacy, of course.

2. My father pointed out that the security guard might have been a *lamedvavnikim*, one of the *tzaddikim*, or Jewish "saints," walking undetected among us. Tradition holds that there are always thirty-six of them on Earth at any given time.

3. National Core Indicators 2018-19 Survey. https://www.nationalcoreindicators.org, retrieved November 24, 2020.

4. Fletcher, R. et al. ed. (2007). Diagnostic Manual-Intellectual Disability: A Clinical Guide for Diagnosis of Mental Disorders in Persons with Intellectual Disability. NADD Press.

5. Ozer, E., Weiss, D. (2004). *Who develops post-traumatic stress disorder?* Current Directions in Psychological Science, 13(4), 169-172.

6. *Crime against persons with disabilities, 2009—2015—Statistical tables. Bureau of Justice Statistics 2017. https://www.bjs.gov/content/pub/pdf/capd0915st.pdf. Retrieved December 11, 2020. According the U.S. Department of Justice statistics, in 2011, 2.7 per 1000 persons with a disability experienced rape or a sexual assault, compared to .9 per 1000 people without a disability; 36.7 per 1,000 experiences some kind of assault compared with 16.7 per 1000 of people without a disability. Researchers estimate that only one out of thirty cases of sexual abuse gets reported. See Harrell, Erika (2017).*

7. Valentini-Hein, D., Schwarts, L. D. (1995). The sexual abuse interview for those with developmental disabilities. James Stanfield Company.

8. *For a concise discussion, see* McGilvery, S. (2018). The identification and treatment of trauma in individuals with developmental disabilities. NADD Press.

9. Sobsey, D. (1994). Violence in the lives of people with disabilities: The end of silent acceptance. Baltimore, MD: P. H. Brooks. *Sobsey is one of the pioneers of addressing how frequently people with I/DD experience trauma.*

10. Kendall, K., Owen, M. (2015). Intellectual Disability and Psychiatric Comorbidity: Challenges and Clinical Issues. *Psychiatric Times*, May 26, 2015, Vol 32 No 5.

11. National Core Indicators 2018-19 Survey. https://www. nationalcoreindicators.org, retrieved November 24, 2020

12. Herman, J. (1992). Trauma and Recovery. Basic Books. *Judith Herman talks at length here about how frequently trauma is misdiagnosed. She highlights bipolar disorder, borderline personality disorder, and schizophrenia as three of the most common misdiagnoses of trauma, though behavior disorders rank highly too. My experience has borne this out. It's hard to overstate how important this book is for understanding trauma. It was the basis of my graduate research and my master's thesis back in 1998, and it was one of the three books I chose as texts for teaching my trauma class twenty years later. At the time of this writing, her book was in its fourteenth printing. For readers who want to learn about the fundamentals of trauma, from its historic beginnings to how we approach treatment today,* Trauma and Recovery *is irreplaceable.*

13. Snowden, L. 2003. Bias in Mental Health Assessment and Intervention: Theory and Evidence. *American Journal of Public Health* 93, 239-243 https://doi.org/10.2105/AJPH.93.2.239.

14. Merino, Y. et al. "Implicit Bias and Mental Health Professionals: Priorities and Directions for Research." *Psychiatric Services*, Vol. 69. Issue 6. June 2018, pp. 723-25.

15. Fadus, M. et al. "Unconscious Bias and the Diagnosis of Disruptive Behavior Disorders and ADHD in African American and Hispanic Youth." *Academic Psychiatry* 44, 95–102 (2020). https://doi.org/10.1007/s40596-019-01127-6.

16. Reiss, S., & Szyszko, J. (1983). *Diagnostic overshadowing and professional experience with mentally retarded persons.* American Journal of Mental Deficiency, 87, 396-402. *Steven Reiss not only coined this term but was fascinated by many topics ranging from temperament to religion. I recommend* Who Am I: 16 Basic Desires That Motivate Our Actions, Define Our Personalities (2000)*, a high point of his later work and a good resource for developing self-awareness.*

17. Deb, S. *The Use of Medication for the Management of Problem (Challenging) Behaviour in Adults who Have Intellectual Disabilities.* University of Hertfordshire, Intellectual Disability and Health. Originally published 2004; revised 2012, 2018. Retrieved April 23, 2021.

18. National Core Indicators 2018-19 Survey. https://www. nationalcoreindicators.org, retrieved November 24, 2020.

19. Hulsman, J. (2018). *To Dare More Boldly: The Audacious Story of Political Risk.* Princeton, NJ: Princeton University Press. *Full disclosure: Hulsman is a personal friend and occasional writing partner. While his political science book may seem like an odd choice to include here, I chose this quote from a chapter devoted to what happens when we refuse to look realistically at our own role in a problem. Spoiler: bad things. This is true whether you're a helping professional or you're the Roman Empire.*

20. *For a longer discussion of the history of the history of behaviorism in I/DD, see this excellent overview at* Parallels in Time: A History of Developmental Disabilities: Part One: The Ancient Era to the 1950s. MN Department of Administration Council on Disabilities. http://mn.govddc/ parallels/index.html.

21. A wise old psychotherapist once said, "Never underestimate how much we can heal by simply living long enough."

22. van der Kolk, B. (2012). *Trauma, Attachment and Neuroscience: New Therapeutic Treatments.* CMI Education Institute webcast, December 14, 2012.

23. *Ibid.*

24. van der Kolk, B. (2015). *The Body Keeps the Score: Brain, Mind and Body in the Healing of Trauma.* New York: Penguin Books.

25. Porges, S. (2011). *The Polyvagal Theory: Neurophysiological Foundations of Emotions, Attachment, Communication, and Self-regulation.* New York: Norton and Co.

26. Siegel, D. (2020). *The Developing Mind: How Relationships and the Brain Interact to Shape Who We Are.* 3rd Ed. New York: Guilford Press.

27. van der Kolk, B. (2015). *The Body Keeps the Score: Brain, Mind and Body in the Healing of Trauma.* New York: Penguin Books.

28. Diagnostic and Statistical Manual of Mental Disorders, 5th ed. American Psychiatric Association. 2013

29. Perry, B. et al. (1995). Childhood trauma, the neurobiology of adaption, and "use-dependent" development of the brain: How "states" become "traits." *Infant Mental Health Journal.* Vol 16, no. 4.

30. van der Kolk, B. (2015). *The Body Keeps the Score: Brain, Mind and Body in the Healing of Trauma.* New York: Penguin Books.

31. Shapiro, F. (2018). *Eye Movement Desensitization and Reprocessing (EMDR) Therapy : Basic Principles, Protocols, and Procedures.* 3rd Ed. New York: The Guilford Press.

32. Sobsey, D. (1994). *Violence in the Lives of People with Disabilities: The End of Silent Acceptance.* Baltimore, MD: P. H. Brooks.

33. National Core Indicators 2018-19 Survey. https://www. nationalcoreindicators.org, retrieved November 24, 2020.

34. American Psychiatric Association (2013). Diagnostic and Statistical Manual of Mental Disorders, 5th ed. *There was heated debate in the writing of the DSM-5 about adding more categories of trauma disorders, including one for children ("developmental trauma disorder"). We may see more diagnostic categories such as that one in future editions.*

35. Gentile, J, et al. (2019). *Guide to Intellectual Disabilities: A Clinical Handbook.* New York: Springer.

36. Gregory Bateson, in Cozolino, L. (2017). *The Neuroscience of Psychotherapy: Healing the Social Brain.* 3rd Ed. New York: Norton and Co. *Here in his essential book about the "social brain," Cozolino quotes British thinker Gregory Bateson, who was talking about the forces that shape us from our beginnings and that determine how we expect things to go for us in the world. Psychotherapy, then, is the process of finding out what we deeply "know" without thinking and then recognizing and challenging those assumptions.*

37. Harvey, K. (2009). *Positive Identity Development: An Alternative Treatment Approach for Individuals with Mild and Moderate Intellectual Disabilities.* Kingston, NY: NADD Press.

38. Barrett, L. (2020). *7½ Lessons About the Brain.* New York: Houghton Mifflin Harcourt.

39. Palay, L. (2017). "The Brain, The Body and the Mind," online chapter

in *Integrative Body Mind Spirit Social Work,* 2nd ed., Lee, et al. Oxford University Press.

40. Cozolino, L. (2017). *The Neuroscience of Psychotherapy: Healing the Social Brain*, 3rd Ed. New York: Norton and Co.

41. van der Kolk, B. (2015). *The Body Keeps the Score: Brain, Mind and Body in the Healing of Trauma.* New York: Penguin Books.

42. Porges, S. (2011). *The Polyvagal Theory: Neurophysiological Foundations of Emotions, Attachment, Communication, and Self-regulation.* New York: Norton and Co.

43. Benson, H. (1984). *Beyond the Relaxation Response.* New York: Berkley Books.

44. *This "safety script" and the example of the ascending card task were shared by the wonderful trauma clinician (and friend of mine) Mary Vicario, LPCC-S, in a presentation of hers that I attended years ago. I've described them here with her kind permission.*

45. Ellingsen, D. et al. The neurobiology shaping affective touch: Expectation, motivation and meaning in the multisensory context. *Frontiers in Psychology*, 6:1986. 2016.

46. G. Dölen et al. Social Reward Requires Coordinated Activity of Nucleus Accumbens Oxytocin and Serotonin. *Nature*, 501, 179-184. 2013.

47. Matthews, G. et al. Dorsal Raphe Dopamine Neurons Represent the Experience of Social Isolation. *Cell*, vol. 164, no. 4. 2016.

48. 1 John 4:18, King James Version: "There is no fear in love; but perfect love casteth out fear: because fear hath torment. He that feareth is not made perfect in love."

49. McGee, J. (1987). *Gentle Teaching: A Nonaversive Approach for Helping Persons with Mental Retardation.* New York: Human Sciences Press. *When I was at the Ohio Department of Developmental Disabilities, I helped to establish the extraordinary John McGee's work in Ohio. I heard him speak not long before his death in 2012, and it was revelatory, but the thing that stood out the most for me was his wry comment that while some people were made uncomfortable by saying it, the simplest word to describe his approach was "love." We should all be so brave.*

50. *Ibid.*

51. *Ibid.*

52. Sobsey, D. (1994). *Violence in the Lives of People with Disabilities: The End of Silent Acceptance.* Baltimore, MD: P. H. Brooks.

53. McGilvery, S. (2018). *The Identification and Treatment of Trauma in Individuals with Developmental Disabilities.* Kingston, NY: NADD Press.

54. "Parallels in Time: A History of Developmental Disabilities: Part One: The Ancient Era to the 1950s." MN Department of Administration Council on Disabilities. http://mn.govddc/parallels/index.html.

55. Aldridge, K. (2020). Personal communication: *Token economies in group settings, behavior management plans/goals, applied behavioral analysis (ABA); the variations are endless. In the early days, when caring for people with disabilities first shifted from the family to state-sponsored care, the focus was almost exclusively custodial. Amid such a limited focus, behavioralist theory was revolutionary. It opened untold possibilities through advancements in teach/training techniques. Unfortunately, the massive success of behavioral approaches in working with people with developmental disabilities may have had some unintended negative side effects. As approaches to treating mental illness and emotional disturbances involved a deeper understanding of the interplay between emotions, thoughts, and actions, behavioral approaches in the I/DD world still tended toward actions, or behaviors, as the dominant factor, almost to the exclusion of the other two. As our understanding of trauma has advanced, we have begun to see the negative impact of such a perspective. A perfect example is the dramatic change over the last decade in our attitudes toward restraints: from useful tools to outmoded and, in many cases, dangerous practices. Our increased caution around actions that may retraumatize a person is a big part of this shift.*

56. O'Dwyer, M. et al. Medication use and potentially inappropriate prescribing in older adults with intellectual disabilities: a neglected area of research. *Therapeutic advances in drug safety*, Vol. 9,9 535-557. Jun. 20 2018

57. Edelsohn G. et al. Psychotropic prescribing for persons with intellectual disabilities and other psychiatric disorders. *Psychiatric Services.* Feb. 1; 65(2):201-7. 2014

58. McLaren, J., & Lichtenstein, J. (2019). The pursuit of the magic pill: The overuse of psychotropic medications in children with intellectual and developmental disabilities in the USA. *Epidemiology and Psychiatric Sciences*, 28 (4), 365-368.

59. Razza, N. and Sobsey, D. (2011). "Treating Survivors of Sexual and Interpersonal Abuse," *Psychotherapy for People with Intellectual Disabilities*. R. Fletcher, Ed. Kingston, NY: NADD Press.

60. Friedman C, Crabb C. Restraint, Restrictive Intervention, and Seclusion of People with Intellectual and Developmental Disabilities. *Intellect Dev Disabil*. Jun 2018;56(3):171-187. doi: 10.1352/1934-9556-56.3.171. PMID: 29782229.

61. Gaskin CJ, McVilly KR, McGillivray JA. Initiatives to reduce the use of seclusion and restraints on people with developmental disabilities: a systematic review and quantitative synthesis. *Res Dev Disabil*. 2013 Nov; 34(11):3946-61. doi: 10.1016/j.ridd.2013.08.010. Epub 2013 Sep 8. PMID: 24025440.

62. *It's hard to find a single statistic to measure restraints and seclusion in the U.S. Data are available for specific populations, and exploring that meaningfully would take too much time here when it's been discussed in other, better ways by many authors. It's also depressingly easy to find numbers of deaths in restraint—they occur every year. There is a wealth of research and documentation that restraint may be impossible to do without risk, and there are a number of organizations pushing for dramatically reducing and eventually eliminating restraint entirely. My reading suggests it's safe to say restraint is decreasing but still happens too often.*

63. Gluckman, P. and Hanson, C. (2006). "Mismatch," Bailey, B. (2014). *Conscious Discipline: Building Resilient Classrooms*. Oviedo, FL: Loving Guidance, Inc.

64. Harvey, K. (2012). *Trauma-Informed Behavioral Interventions: What Works and What Doesn't*. Silver Spring: MD: American Association of Intellectual and Developmental Disabilities. *Harvey, a psychologist with decades of experience designing and working with behavior plans, has written and spoken at length about the limitations of a purely behavioral mindset when it comes to trauma and people with I/DD. Full disclosure: I am also happy to count her as a friend.*

65. Yalom, I. (1989). *Love's Executioner and Other Tales of Psychotherapy.* New York: Basic Books. *Irvin Yalom was one of the most influential authors I read in school. A giant in existential psychotherapy, his work formed much of how I think about working with people, and this lovely quote of his is something I use whenever I get the chance.*

66. van der Kolk, B. (2015). *The Body Keeps the Score: Brain, Mind and Body in the Healing of Trauma.* New York: Penguin Books.

67. Winnicott, D.W. (1971). *Playing and Reality.* Devon, UK: Tavistock Publications.

68. Johnson, S. (2005). *The Practice of Emotionally Focused Couple Therapy: Creating Connection*, 2nd ed. New York: Routledge Press.

69. Bailey, B. (2014). *Conscious Discipline: Building Resilient Classrooms.* Oveido, FL: Loving Guidance, Inc.

70. *Ibid.*

71. Siegel, D. (2007). *The Mindful Brain: Reflection and Attunement in the Cultivation of Well-Being.* New York: Norton and Co.

72. Epstein, M. (1999). *Going to Pieces Without Falling Apart: A Buddhist Perspective on Wholeness.* New York: Harmony.

About the Author

Lara Palay, LISW-S is a psychotherapist with twenty-five years in private practice, specializing in trauma and loss. A co-founder of Aldridge Palay Consulting, Ms. Palay started her career as an hourly worker in the mental health field and went on to be a supervisor and clinical director for multiple mental health agencies. In addition to clinical practice, she has taught social work graduate students for more than a decade. Ms. Palay served as the project manager for the Mental Illness and Developmental Disabilities Coordinating Center of Excellence for the state of Ohio, helping to advance trauma awareness in dual diagnosis. A graduate of The Ohio State University, Ms. Palay lives with her husband and a random assortment of spoiled pets.

www.ingramcontent.com/pod-product-compliance
Lightning Source LLC
Chambersburg PA
CBHW070345270326
41926CB00017B/3992